JUST LET GO!

Achieving health, wellness, and a balanced life

JUST LET GO!

Achieving health, wellness, and a balanced life

LEANNE TOLLEY

BONNEVILLE
SPRINGVILLE, UTAH

This is not an official publication of The Church of Jesus Christ of Latter-day Saints. The opinions and views expressed herein belong solely to the author and do not necessarily represent the opinions or views of Cedar Fort, inc. Permission for the use of sources, graphics, and photos is also solely the responsibility of the author.

ISBN 13: 978-1-59955-439-6

Published by Bonneville Books, an imprint of Cedar Fort, Inc., 2373 W. 700 S., Springville, UT 84663

Distributed by Cedar Fort, Inc., www.cedarfort.com

LIBRARY OF CONGRESS CATALOGING-IN-PUBLICATION DATA
Tolley, LeAnne, 1965-
  Just let go! / LeAnne Tolley.
     p. cm.
  ISBN 978-1-59955-439-6
  1. Psychological literature--United States. 2. Yoga--Therapeutic use. 3. Yoga--Psychological aspects. 4. Self-help techniques--United States. 5. Success--United States--Psychological aspects. I. Title.

B132.Y6T66 2010
181'.45--dc22

2010025640

Cover design by Danie Romrell
Cover design © 2010 by Lyle Mortimer
Edited and typeset by Megan E. Welton

Printed in the United States of America

10 9 8 7 6 5 4 3 2 1

Printed on acid-free paper

There are so many people who have made this book a reality that I can't begin to thank them all personally.

To my family and friends for not laughing at me for thinking I could actually write a book;

To my students for their unwavering belief that I really had something worthwhile to say;

To my kids for treating me like a celebrity;

And, finally,

To my husband for all the late nights in the hot tub just listening to ME when you could have been listening to your MP3 player!

CONTENTS

INTRODUCTION

S EVERAL YEARS AGO, I WAS ASKED TO SPEAK ABOUT
body image issues at a regional women's confer-
ence. I had done this many times before, and that
day, I jokingly stated that maybe I should compile my
research and notes into a book. At the end of my pre-
sentation, a young woman approached me and asked
if I was serious about writing a book. I told her, yes, I
was serious but I didn't know exactly where to start.
She handed me her business card and replied that when
I was ready, she worked for a publisher and would love
to be a part of my project.

I misplaced her business card, but the desire to
put my notes and thoughts into a tangible offering
has stayed with me since that day. I have finally made
room in my life to accomplish this goal and, wouldn't
you know it, I found that business card.

You might be expecting a yoga book to be a simple
instruction manual on poses and postures—well, this

one isn't. I am saving that for my next work. This book focuses on the other 80 percent of yoga—the mind/spirit practices of awareness, mindfulness, and true whole-being connection. If you are looking at yoga merely to fulfill an "exercise" need in your life, you have missed the entire essence of the practice.

The word "yoga" means to "yoke together" the mind, body, and spirit into a well-connected partnership to embrace life! Physical movement is important, but it is only a small part of the wealth of knowledge yoga has to offer. I have plenty to write about my personal approach to the physical aspects of yoga—I plan to do that in the near future—but I believe the true benefit of these physical postures can only be found once we have created a solid, mindful foundation.

This book is dedicated to helping build that foundation. It will ask many soul-searching questions that only you have the answers to. This book is not about "spoon-feeding" you my concept of how to answer life's challenging questions; rather, it's about waking you up so that you can find your own answers—to challenge you to start thinking and questioning for yourself.

For many years, I have worked with eating disorder patients. I have used various yoga principles of mind–body–spirit connection as an experiential therapy for recovery. In my work with body image issues and eating disorders, I always come back to the same starting point—somewhere along the way, we became disconnected from ourselves.

We have created one world for our minds to reside in and a different world for our bodies to reside in. The struggle comes from trying to force our bodies to conform to the world our minds live in. Typically, the world of the mind resides somewhere outside of the present moment. We spend our early years concentrating on the future and our later years contemplating the past. Where are the years devoted to today?

I began writing specifically to address eating disorders but soon came to realize that this mind-body disconnect is pervasive throughout our entire society. As I work with families of eating disorder patients, I see many of the same body image issues, to a lesser degree, manifest in many of them—they just can't see it. We have become so far removed from conscious living that we are unable to connect to what we say and feel in any given moment. There is so much "therapy" all around us that simply concentrates on an individual's victimization—what has happened to us or mistakes or choices we have made—instead of focusing on an individual's ability to change regardless of personal history.

We are so caught up with analyzing the past that we can't exist in the present. Most of our brain function is taken up with questions of "What have I done?" or "What am I going to do?" We rarely connect to the question "What am I doing right now?" This book is an attempt to help clarify the reasons behind this disconnect from which so many of us suffer and to offer useful techniques to create and improve the mind-body-spirit connection.

As I became more aware of this disconnect among the families I was working with, I also noticed these same characteristics showing up among students in all my yoga classes. Regardless of the population I was teaching, the same negative body issues kept coming up over and over again. It felt like an epidemic, but everyone seemed to instinctively embrace instead of fight!

We are constantly bombarded with images, advertisements, and experts who tell us we are not good enough and that we must change. We are told to become masters of our bodies and quit being lazy. As we engage in this role of master, we place our bodies in the role of slave, and we actually seem to enjoy throwing the slave into the ring with the lions—just like they did in ancient times! Before long, I recognized the need for a positive, gentle, uplifting voice in the arena.

I discovered that my students needed permission to actually like themselves again! I decided it was time for a revolution of reconnection.

This all sounds well and good, but to what purpose? I hope this book will move beyond the "self-help" label to a place of stronger impact. I hope it serves as a "true-self" book. After all, what's the use of self-help if it isn't to aid us in becoming better acquainted with our true selves?

Whatever our goals may be, we will only be happy with achieving them if these goals support and enhance our true selves. In other words we must reconnect with our own intuition, take back responsibility, and find our own voice. This reconnect will allow us to embrace life fully and move beyond ourselves to enhance the world around us.

My husband finds it ironic that this entire book is about "connection," yet the title is about letting go. I try to explain to him that, just like many other phrases, letting go can mean totally different things to different people at different times.

"Just let go" can be interpreted in so many ways. If we are full of tension and stress, it can be an invitation to relax and renew—to permit ourselves to get rid of anxiety and activity. If we are couch potatoes, however, it can be an encouragement to get out of our comfort zone—to jump out of the airplane and sky dive! Think about riding your bike without holding the handlebars. Do you remember ever saying, "Look, Ma! No hands!"? This type of letting go is far different from lying down and relaxing.

Letting go can be relaxing or invigorating; it all depends on the moment. The only way to recognize what the moment will require is to be present, open, and available. Get ready to be challenged, and when you're ready—just let go!

1 | STEPPING INTO STILLNESS: MY STORY

I WAS THE SHORT, CHUBBY ONE. I NEVER REALLY gave my size much thought until I was in high school, where I started noticing a preoccupation with weight among my friends. Fad diets were everywhere. One friend ate so many carrots that her skin became orange-tinged. During this time, I became self-conscious about my body in a way that I had never experienced before. Maybe this is due to the fact that I was a "late bloomer." I tried different diets, such as eating only one meal a day or eating only grapefruit. The diets never helped me lose weight; they merely made me impossible to live with.

In college, I took an aerobics class, and it felt as if a lightbulb had turned on in my brain. I loved it! I felt strong and alive, and I was finally able to achieve a positive attitude toward my body. I recognized that I would never be a tall, thin model, but I could be a strong and active "me." I also enrolled in a fencing class, which gave me a feeling of grace and fluidity that I had never felt before. I was on the right track.

Shortly after college, I was married and living in Seattle. I decided to become a certified aerobics instructor to help other women, like myself, embrace their bodies and avoid wishing they were someone else. I taught many different classes, including step aerobics, which was the newest trend in exercise at the time. I found a deep connection to teaching and encouraging women to identify with their bodies and enjoyed watching my students discover the amazing aspects of feeling positive about their bodies.

Body image is a compilation of personal feelings toward your body that are influenced by external factors such as family, friends, media, work, and so on. Individual body image is reflected in our acceptance and judgment of our own bodies in comparison to others, either those around us or images in the media. We express our body image to the world through our words and actions, such as criticizing our bodies and displaying poor posture.

Interestingly enough, we feel as if negative body image is a good thing. None of us wants to be thought of as conceited, so we feel more comfortable speaking critically about ourselves—usually in the hopes that others will tell us that what we say is not true. This cycle of negative talk, followed by the need for others to deny our words, soon becomes a habit of negative body image. We tend to continue hearing our own words of negativity while ignoring the positive words of others.

I found this cycle to be prevalent among the students in my aerobics classes. Class would usually start with students trickling in and conversing with each other. The typical comments would be "I hope we are going to work on legs today—I hate my thighs." Or, "I hate my stomach—I need to do more ab work." I rarely heard a positive comment about attending class; instead, it was always about hating something and wanting to fix it—NOW! There was also an overwhelming feeling of "duty" to attend class in order to demand that the student's body become something other than what it was to start with. Students often had looks of intense concentration and determination as they moved through the routines; there were very few facial expressions of enjoyment.

Many of the teachers that I worked with incorporated a philosophy of recognizing improvement but never being satisfied. They would encourage their students to always seek for more physical change and to worry about "backsliding." I felt it was my responsibility as a teacher to change this attitude towards body image. I wanted to instill a sense of connection and excitement within my students rather than just a hard workout and a drive for more.

By this time, I had moved to Utah, and I began teaching with a more holistic purpose. I wanted to create a safe environment for every student, not just the really active and fit participants. I felt that those who were less active were the students who really needed to feel welcome in an exercise facility so they would continue to be active.

I didn't want my students to feel like I was in competition with them or that I always had to be superior to their abilities. I wanted to really teach them something about themselves that maybe they wouldn't learn anywhere else. I offered modifications and alternatives to those who needed them and more advanced techniques to others. I wanted my classes to be appropriate and available to all levels of fitness. I wanted to *teach*, not just instruct.

I soon got the reputation of being the "nice" teacher—the one who would encourage students to push themselves rather than demand they keep up with me. Other aerobics instructors would refer some of their students to my classes—new students who weren't keeping up or who weren't looking for a "knock-down, drag-out" class. At first, I was upset: did they think I wasn't a good teacher? Did they think I wasn't able to teach the hard stuff? Did they think I couldn't be as tough as they were? I questioned what I was doing.

I found a need within my students and addressed

this need when others didn't. I realized there were a lot more beginners than experts, and these students needed a teacher who could help them get started. I also noticed a change of dialog in my classes. Instead of comments about hating their bodies, students would ask me if we were going to practice a certain routine because they really liked how it made them feel. I was witnessing the change in their personal awareness of themselves—their body image—and I wasn't going to give this up for anything! My classes were becoming what I had always imagined—a place to connect the mind, body, and spirit. I was making a difference. At the same time, I was also experiencing great physical pain.

In 1988, I had injured my left shoulder and was diagnosed with a shoulder separation. I was in a shoulder brace for six weeks and unable to do my normal exercise routines. I heard someone at the gym talking about yoga, so I looked into doing a few stretching exercises to strengthen my shoulder. It helped a little, and I liked the movements, but I was attached to my aerobics classes, so I didn't really give yoga a second thought.

Five years later, I continued to have shoulder problems, and they were getting progressively worse. I attributed the pain to arthritis, which, according to my doctor, was a common occurrence with shoulder separation injuries. My husband finally convinced me to see another doctor about the problem. After months of tests administered by multiple doctors, I was diagnosed with a sterno-clavicular separation. At the time of my shoulder injury, my clavicle (collar bone) had separated from my sternum also. The doctors informed me that surgery would be necessary to save the movement in my left arm and to repair the damage to my sternum, clavicle, and neck muscles.

Because of the rarity of the injury, there was only one doctor in Utah who would be able to perform surgery, and I was immediately referred to Dr. Sherman S. Coleman at the University of Utah Medical Center. The surgery took place in November of 1993, and I was again in a shoulder and neck brace for three months.

Among other reconstructions, the surgery required the removal of a portion of my left clavicle at the sternal end, leaving the bone "floating," as the doctor described. I was told that I would probably never again be able to go water skiing, rock climbing, or take part in any other form of exercise that required tension of the clavicle for support—not even pushups. *But wait*, I thought, *I'm an aerobics teacher!* How was this going to be possible? I felt lost.

Fortunately, I was able to return to teaching in early 1994, but it wasn't the same. I had lost much of the upper body strength I relied on to teach. I was diminished physically and mentally. I needed a new approach to life. I took a leave of absence from teaching aerobics and focused on recovery. I joined a different gym and took both aerobics and yoga classes on a regular basis. While I still enjoyed the aerobics classes, the yoga classes were helping my body heal and adjust to its new limitations.

At first, I was worried—would yoga be against my personal belief system? Isn't yoga tied to specific religions? Is this an acceptable activity—especially in a state like Utah? I decided that I needed to learn more about what yoga is and—more importantly—what yoga isn't.

I researched the philosophy of yoga and found that, just like anything else, you can find someone to support just about any side of the argument. There are many people who feel that you can't practice yoga *and* be a good Christian. There are many people who feel that you can't be a good yoga practitioner if you aren't of the Hindu belief system. The double-sided list went on and on.

The more I studied, the more I came to believe that yoga is uniquely suited to support anyone in his own personal belief system and that it doesn't require anyone to conform to a specific set of religious beliefs; rather, it merely encourages the individual to embrace his specific set of personal beliefs. Things like "non-stealing," "non-greed," "purity," and "self-study," among many others, are all part of the yoga philosophy.

I found that yoga truly enhanced my spiritual growth within my own belief system. It also gave me a good kick in the pants, reminding me to be constantly mindful about what I believe.

I found, though, that many of the classes offered in the gyms were what I would call aerobic yoga, or "aeroga"—which is my nickname for these classes. They focused on doing yoga postures from an aerobic mindset. There was no connection between what we were doing and what we were feeling. Pushing our bodies to their ultimate limits—and sometimes beyond—seemed to be a trend in many of the yoga classes at the gyms. This wasn't really what I understood yoga to be.

I soon realized that I wanted to do more than just participate in yoga classes, I wanted to teach. I attended every yoga workshop I could find and eventually decided that I needed to research what training was required to become a traditional or authentic yoga teacher.

I then began teaching yoga classes, incorporating what I was learning from the workshops and other traditional yoga classes. I was teaching at the gym as well as offering a free community class twice a week. I was building a strong teaching foundation, but I finally decided that I needed to have more formal training.

I found a four-month teacher training program with Nancy Ruby, the founder of YogaMotion™

in Bozeman, Montana. What drew me to Nancy's program was the incorporation of various forms and methods of yoga as well as the intense focus on anatomy and physiology. This program reinforced the foundation for my teaching philosophy.

I felt an immediate connection between my personal teaching philosophy and the holistic approaches within a deeper exploration of yoga. Nancy focused on recognizing the uniqueness of the individual and being present while we are on the mat. She reinforced the concept of making choices that are right for us in the moment—to connect with what is happening. Nancy taught us to turn off the external noise and listen to our own internal dialog. She reinforced the need for teachers to be willing to experience what their students are feeling and to exist from the inside out. This was the teaching style I had always wanted to embrace. The lightbulb got brighter.

Nancy also reminded us to not be offended by the fact that not every student will like every teacher and to remember that the reverse is also true. Teachers and students will eventually find their way to one another. They will be drawn to personalities and styles that will make the most of their experience. She taught us that above all, we should teach from a place of honesty—to offer who we really are.

Nancy tried to instill in us the concept that there are plenty of students just waiting for our individual and unique teaching style, and they will find us when we are ready to teach. Those who don't fit with our style will slowly move toward other teachers, and those who are inspired by our style will bring other students to join us. I reflected back on my insecurities as an aerobics teacher and realized that I had learned this concept earlier and now needed to embrace it fully.

Nancy explained that beginners are the hardest group to teach. Those who are already "experts" in any given arena don't really need expert teachers. All they need is minimal guidance—someone to call out the moves. It is the beginning student that needs the most experienced teacher to create a safe, welcoming, and appropriate environment. The hardest thing to create is the foundation, but this step is the most important.

These philosophies seemed to encourage me as a teacher and support the path that I was traveling. At the same time that I was studying with Nancy Ruby, I was asked to teach yoga classes at The Center for Change (CFC or The Center). CFC is an inpatient facility for girls with eating disorders (commonly referred to as ED). One of the other teachers at the gym was also working as a dietician at CFC and thought my teaching style would fit well with the patients.

I was excited about the prospect of working with students who really needed new insights to body image issues. Most of the patients were obsessive about exercise and tended to overexercise to the point of injury. I knew that yoga—and, perhaps, my teaching style—could offer a new perspective to exercise and what it means to be actively healthy.

As I worked with the patients at CFC, I recognized a change in my own attitude toward being actively healthy. I was no longer concerned with limitations to my shoulder and was finding that if I really listened and connected with my body I was able to alter and modify movements to build strength again. I was able to do push-ups when utilizing yoga techniques, and I achieved full range of motion—something I never thought possible. As I relearned how to connect within my own body, I was able to share these lessons with the students I was teaching at CFC, at the gym, and in the community.

My teaching became more meaningful to me and to my students. I started defining "life lessons" within the practice. I made connections between attitudes on the mat to attitudes off the mat. I was no longer simply teaching postures—I was teaching life skills. I began teaching in various facilities around the valley and started offering personal lessons from my home. I continued to attend workshops and training, started training new yoga teachers, and offered workshops of my own.

As a result of my work at CFC and my other classes, I received requests to speak to various groups;

from high school and college classes to community, religious, and civic groups. I compiled binders of research information and personal experience notes for these speaking engagements. I focused on body image issues and the importance of the mind-body-spirit connection. While I tailored my comments to different audiences, I found that a continuous theme was apparent in every presentation I gave—the lack of mind-body-spirit connection was prevalent in any given demographic.

While I had been teaching yoga for many years, I became a traditionally certified yoga teacher in 2002. In 2004, I became a nationally registered yoga teacher through Yoga Alliance. I have continued to study and train in additional yoga areas and have specialized in anatomy and physiology as well as energy and chakra work.

So now my goal in every teaching and speaking opportunity is the same—to identify, explain, and encourage life practices that will build upon the connection between the mind, the body, and the spirit without creating a hard-line definition of these concepts. Each individual is unique, and so is his definition of these three areas. My goal as a teacher and speaker is to create a safe, comfortable, general concept and then allow the student to refine the idea to complement his circumstance.

Through years of teaching and speaking about

body image issues, I have reflected back on my experience as an aerobics instructor. I recognize now that the strong attachment to aerobics stemmed from my initial experience as the "short, chubby one." The rapid movements of aerobics—step aerobics in particular—allowed me to turn off the voice in my head that repeated that phrase so consistently.

When I started practicing yoga, I had to create moments of stillness. All of a sudden, I heard that voice again. This time, though, I was prepared with skills to cope with the voice, and I opened a new dialog with that short, chubby one that created a new sense of acceptance and enjoyment. I loved teaching aerobics. I loved teaching weight lifting. I loved teaching all the other types of exercise classes that I taught.

Just because I teach yoga doesn't mean that I think it is the only thing everyone should do—I just know that it is right for me right now. Some days, I really feel like lifting weights, so I do. Some days, I really feel like swimming, so I do. Some days, I really feel like riding a bike, so I do. It is not about what we do, it is about why we do it. It is about being honest with ourselves and our motives. We need to do what we love—when we love it. And we need to allow it to change with our changing life.

I have moved from step aerobics to yoga. I have stepped into stillness. I'm still probably short—depending on whom I stand next to. I'm still probably chubby—depending on whom I stand next to. But now that short, chubby one has a name, just like all short, chubby ones do, and her name is LeAnne.

2 | EMBRACING LIFE AS A SKI COAT

THE MIND-BODY-SPIRIT CONNECTION IS OFTEN DE-
scribed as being similar to a hand inside a glove.
The body is compared to the glove, and the hand is
compared to the mind-spirit component, which gives
the body animation. This comparison seems to lack
the true essence of life. It is too easy to put the two
together or take the two apart. There is no true con-
nectivity in this example. It leaves a feeling of distinc-
tion and separation at all times.

Instead, the mind-body-spirit connection is more
similar to a ski coat. There is a lightweight, water-
proof outer shell and a warm, substantial inner shell.
To use the two parts together, they are first connected
with the snaps at the wrist and neck. Then the entire
lining is zipped to the outer shell. The outer and inner
shells are now dependent on each other to form one
coat that meets multiple needs.

These points of actual connection are what help the separate coats work together and feel more comfortable. It takes work to both combine the two and take the two apart. The connections are necessary to fulfill the ultimate purpose of the coat.

At times, these connections can be uncomfortable. While teaching a class in reflexology at CFC one afternoon, one of the patients stated that she hated to touch her hands and feet. This caught me by surprise, so I questioned her about this attitude. "I don't like to think about what's in there," she stated. "It grosses me out to feel inside." This idea confused me, especially because this patient loves shoes, so it couldn't be a feeling of dislike for her feet in general. "I can look at them from the outside, but I don't want to have to think about them from the inside," was her reply.

The concept of experiencing our body from the outside-in is typical of modern society. By removing an internal sense of connection, society is able to create a desire for cookie-cutter conformity. Individuals try to become what they see, not what they instinctively feel. People learn to ignore what is happening inside in favor of what is going on around them. The intuitive voice is silenced in an effort to be part of the external world.

So, where does this disconnect begin? Why does it even matter? It begins with the elimination of attention to the senses. By ignoring other senses to focus specifically on sight, it becomes easy to ignore the natural inclination toward intuition or instinct.

The world around us is primarily directed toward our sense of vision. From printed media to television and film, visual focus is oversaturated to the detriment of our other senses. Complicating this issue is a lack of visual literacy. Even though the eye takes information in, it is unable to discern the truth of what is seen. Images are manipulated and distorted to create a perfect "mold."

Then the media requires conformation to this distorted mold. People buy into the "one size fits all" approach to life. If someone is successful at a particular business, exercise, or diet, everyone else thinks they should have success the exact same way. By eliminating individuality and intuition, the ability to thrive is diminished. Some individuals need only a few hours of sleep. For those who require more sleep, it can be irritating to be told that it is just a matter of self-control and habits. Of course, it isn't only self-control and habit that determine the need for sleep. Each person is hardwired differently. Individual needs are as unique and diverse as individual brains. If brains are so different, then why is it so easy to buy into the idea that all bodies should look and interact alike? This quest to all look alike leads to negative body image.

The most important issue concerning body image

is the effect that negative body image has on health. When individuals suffer from body dissatisfaction, they tend to look to every available external source for answers. They try to re-create themselves in the image of those who they identify as being happy, successful, and powerful.

Think of it this way. A parent's job is to teach children certain motor skills. Small children are taught which hand is their right and which is their left. The parent says the words and shows the correct response. Then parents say the words without showing the response in order to teach children the connection by words alone. Children learn to see and feel the appropriate response. When asked to show their left or right hand, they connect the words with the internal feeling they have created of left and right.

The concept of feeling the left and right side of the body is rarely used again as adults. The connection between verbal directions that trigger internal awareness is lost. Instead, the world is navigated by pointing at objects or by mirroring and mimicking. Adults have a hard time doing something new unless they actually see someone else do it first. Some of the connection to the sense of sound is lost in exchange for a greater dependence on the sense of sight. A great example of this is the communication of driving directions. Think about it—do people naturally use terms like "north," "south," "left," and "right"? Or do they use visual references such as buildings and hand gestures?

It is easy to test this theory—just ask someone to place his right hand on his left shoulder and watch as he has to stop and think about where he is in space. He's lost that internal feeling of left and right. Individuals become so disconnected from where they are in space that simple actions can't be done without looking around for confirmation of accuracy.

So, how do we reconnect to natural intuition? Better yet, how can the prevalent attitudes that foster mind-body-spirit disconnect be avoided? It's a difficult question to answer.

Many studies have shown that the earlier an emphasis on intuitive living is created, the better the foundation for body image. The first step is to define what is meant by body image. "Body image has been defined as the concept of one's body formed by past and present perceptual and sensory experiences and an experiential reservoir of experiences, affects, and memories."[1]

Body image is determined, in large part, by the connection between the internal self and the external world. People abuse their bodies because they lack a strong connection to what is happening inside. Participating in activities that focus on listening to internal cues is important to overcoming negative body image. The practices encompassed within yoga are uniquely suited to create a "reconnect" between the mind, body, and spirit.

While the use of yoga has been proven to be an effective tool for recovery from eating disorders and negative body image, a more important issue may be the use of yoga as a preventive measure to eliminate the onset of negative body image. In other words, creating a strong foundation to begin with is always better than repairing a weak foundation in the future.

Melinda Scime and Catherine Cook-Cottone address the idea of preventing underlying causes of poor body image that may lead to eating disorders. They lay out the concept of providing young adolescent girls with learning experiences that support the creation of positive body image and turn the focus away from external body awareness to internal body connectedness. These learning experiences may include yoga, discussion of media images, meditation techniques, and mind-body integration awareness.

The study consisted of seventy-five female participants in the fifth grade. Participants filled out questionnaires at the beginning of the study, at regular intervals, and at the end of the study. The questionnaire consisted of items from the standard body dissatisfaction scale, drive for thinness scale, bulimia scale, and many others.

The researchers collected data on the change in answers over the span of the study and found that while discussion of media images and content helped to educate participants about body stereotypes, the greatest factor in diminishing negative body image came from teaching mind-body connection skills to help decrease personal body dissatisfaction. This, in turn, helped to decrease the potential for disordered eating behaviors in the future.

This study identified the positive effects of yoga in decreasing body dissatisfaction and minimizing the effects of the media on body image creation. Early education and positive body image creation are essential to preventing body dissatisfaction and creating healthy body awareness. "If body dissatisfaction can be effectively targeted via interventions aimed at preadolescent females . . . it may protect against the later development of eating disorder attitudes and behaviors."[2]

The yoga practices of meditation and mindfulness help individuals increase awareness of circumstances in any given moment. These tools help individuals focus on what is happening inside as well as outside and offer a reference point for making wise personal decisions that prevent negative body image.

Jennifer Daubenmeir conducted a study of this theory, which involved the participation of three separate groups: yoga students who were not currently taking aerobics classes, aerobics students who were not currently taking yoga classes, and a control group of individuals who had not taken either type of class in the last two years. All three groups completed surveys titled "Women and Exercise" at the beginning of the study. Each question on the survey required an answer on a sliding scale of variables—ranking answers to questions on a scale from one to ten. Daubenmeir found that "the yoga participants reported significantly greater body awareness, responsiveness, body satisfaction, and less self-objectification than the aerobic and baseline groups. . . . For disordered eating attitudes, the yoga group reported lower scores compared to the aerobics group."[3]

Daubenmeir's study confirmed the theory that yoga practitioners experienced a more positive attitude toward their bodies than either the aerobic exercise group or the control group. The yoga group reported less self-objectification and greater satisfaction with their physical appearance. The aerobic exercise group, on the other hand, reported a heightened critical attitude toward their physical appearance—even though participants were selected so that each individual's BMI (body mass index) was considered nearly identical for all groups. In other words, all participants of the study were of similar body size and shape.

> In addition, the concept of body awareness was expanded from its original version proposed by Fredrickson and Roberts (1997) into two aspects: degree of perceptual awareness of internal bodily sensations and degree of responsiveness to them. As expected, yoga practitioners reported both greater awareness and responsiveness. In turn, the greater body responsiveness reported by the yoga participants explained their

less self-objectification, greater body satisfaction, and fewer disordered eating attitudes compared to the non-yoga participants.[4]

Daubenmeir recognizes the importance of body awareness and responsiveness in creating and maintaining positive body image. This awareness is essential in the prevention and elimination of eating disorders and negative body image.

This focus on preventive education is critical as body image issues become more prevalent and symptomatic in our current culture. The increase in the instances of depression may be, in part, attributable to the increase in body dissatisfaction and eating disorders. In a research study published in 2007 by Oxford Journal, Dr. David Shapiro and colleagues studied the positive effects of yoga as a complementary treatment for depression.

This study focused on seventeen participants who were taking medication for depression but were still suffering symptoms. Shapiro collected data such as blood pressure and heart rate before and after classes, and so forth. Participants completed questionnaires that asked for rankings of various answers on a sliding scale.

Yoga practice was shown to decrease negative mood and anxiety and increase feelings of well-being and tranquility among test subjects. These effects were attributed to the use of deep breathing techniques combined with movements that stretched and strengthened the entire body. According to Shapiro, mood changes are central in depression and mood disorders and, therefore, yoga was shown to be a positive therapy for many core issues concerning depression. While participating in yoga movements such as "stretching, balancing, and breathing routines, subjects reported being less anxious, tense, angry, fatigued, and confused after classes than just before class."[5]

Shapiro went on to state that the most significant improvements were reported by those participants who suffered more strongly from depression and anxiety. Shapiro concludes;

> For all who completed the study, aside from clinical symptoms of depression, reductions were also observed in measures of anxiety, expression of anger, neurotic symptoms, limitations on usual role activities because of emotional difficulties. . . . Thus, participation in yoga did not in effect target depression only but also affected psychological and biological processes indicative of improved mental health in general and more effective social behavior.[6]

The use of yoga to prevent body dissatisfaction tendencies, reduce depression symptoms, and rehabilitate eating disorder issues has become a primary focus for well-being. Dorothy Foltz-Gray (2006) identifies yoga as an essential tool to empower women as they seek healthy lifestyles.

In her article, "Happy in Your Own Skin," Foltz-Gray shares the stories of various women and the effect that yoga has had on each of their lives. The first story identifies the concerns of a young woman struggling through puberty and the changes in her body. She speaks of the emotional pain and suffering she experienced during high school and college. The woman then talks about the first time she decided to attend a yoga class and the changes in her attitude and self-identification due to engaging in the practice of yoga.

"I was so nervous that I wouldn't fit in or be able to do the poses and that the other students would have tiny, perfect bodies. . . . But when I walked in, I saw a whole range of people."[7] The young woman started feeling stronger and more comfortable within her body, and the negative voice in her head grew quiet. Foltz-Gray states that what the woman experienced was the beginning of the positive body image process.

"She's among millions of Americans—most of them women—who struggle each day with feelings of shame and inadequacy about their physical selves. . . . Yoga makes a difference because of its emphasis on self acceptance, something that's largely missing for those of us who dislike our bodies."[8]

Another young woman suffered from breast cancer and the physical effects of undergoing a mastectomy and reconstructive surgery. The aftermath of the surgeries left the patient with multiple scars, a diminished body image, and depression. She found it hard to even look at her body in the mirror. Her introduction to yoga allowed her to move away from the visual impact of the surgeries and concentrate on the dynamic power of her body and the ability to create a positive body image by focusing within and then moving outward.

"It was so right here, right now. . . . I could just be in the body I had. I was focusing on my breath and my joints and the muscles I was stretching, not on my upper arm that I hated. . . . I thought, 'This is powerful.' "[9]

Foltz-Gray explains this phenomenon: "What she discovered in her very first class was something wholly unexpected: a profound shift in the way it felt to inhabit her scarred, altered body."[10]

Finally, Foltz-Gray discusses one young woman's struggle to overcome anorexia nervosa. She attended a yoga class because her mother "thought it might allow her to befriend the body she'd abused for so long."[11] The young woman shares the way her yoga teacher created a mindful awareness of her amazing body that she had never experienced before.

> My instructor would start the class talking about what an amazing structure the foot is, how it roots us to the earth. Then she would guide a self-massage of the

foot and encourage us to revel in each sensation. . . . [The teacher] asked us to be conscious of how it felt to walk down the street . . . and to recognize the small miracle of walking. All of that allowed me to think of my body not as something that needed to be changed or that had to be punished but as a vessel that could carry me through anything.[12]

The author concludes with the power of yoga. "Yoga is all about coming into the moment and seeing ourselves as we are. Instead of wishful thinking or putting on an image we want other people to see, in yoga we get still and quiet, and all that falls away."[13]

These stories point to the idea that yoga is not a cure for everything; rather, it's merely a way to become more connected to the inner self, therefore allowing that connection to be more important than a mirror. The underlying message of all of this research is the concept of introducing tools that will help create and support positive body image.

Printed in the Journal of Clinical Child Psychology in 1980, "Body Cathexis in Children as a Function of Awareness Training and Yoga" reports the study of the effects of yoga as an awareness tool to improve body image in a group of third-graders.

The intimate relationship between mind and body suggests that one's body image may strongly affect one's self image. Twelve third-year elementary school students, ten girls and two boys, who demonstrated low body satisfaction and poor physical co-ordination, were randomly assigned to either an experimental group, which received awareness training and yoga exercise, or to a control group.[14]

The study participants were moved from their regular PE classes during school and practiced awareness exercises and yoga instead. The study found that simple yoga therapies, such as mindful movement of hands and feet, were very effective in decreasing dissatisfaction with those particular body areas. The findings also showed an increased desire on the part of the experimental group to participate in activities with the rest of their classmates and a decreased feeling of self-consciousness during physical activity.

Notice the students weren't excluded from doing other forms of activity for the rest of the school year. They were merely offered an alternative class for part of the year and then reintroduced into their regular exercise classes. The newfound optimism and mindfulness, which they learned from the yoga classes, helped create a lasting positive impact on their interaction with their classmates and improved their participation in all forms of exercise and activity.

During a follow-up with the original study participants six months later, researchers discovered an interesting side effect from the introduction of yoga as a body awareness technique. All of the participants were found to have improved their class scores in every area. The positive effects of introducing yoga as a therapeutic tool to improve body image seemed to be pervasive throughout the participants' lives.[15]

While the research itself may be boring, all of the studies seem to support the same idea—the stronger the emphasis placed on creating a solid mind–body-spirit connection, the more secure and positive the feelings of individual body image. When attention is placed on the internal voice, the ski coat can be zipped together to face any storm!

NOTES

1. Pauline Rose Clance, Michael Mitchell, and Suzanne R. Engelman, "Body Cathexis in Children as a Function of Awareness Training and Yoga," *Journal of Child Psychology*, Spring 1980, 82.

2. Melinda Scime and Catherine Cook-Cottone, "Primary Prevention of Eating Disorders: A Constructivist Integration of Mind and Body Strategies," *International Journal of Eating Disorders* 41, no. 2 (2008): 134–42, doi:10.102/eat.

3. Jennifer J. Daubenmeir, "The Relationship of Yoga, Body Awareness, and Body Responsiveness to Self-Objectification and Disordered Eating." *Psychology of Women Quarterly*, 29 (2005): 207–12.

4. Ibid.

5. David Shapiro, Ian A. Cook, Dmitry M. Davydov, Cristina Ottaviani, Andrew F. Leuchter, and Michelle Abrams, "Yoga as a Complementary Treatment of Depression: Effects of Traits and Moods on Treatment Outcome," *OxfordJournal.org Advance Access Publication eCAM* 4, no. 4 (2007): 495.

6. Ibid., 496.

7. Dorothy Foltz-Gray, "Happy in Your Own Skin," *Yoga Journal* 196 (2006): 76.
8. Ibid.
9. Ibid., 77.
10. Ibid.
11. Ibid., 78.
12. Ibid.
13. Ibid.
14. Clance, 83.
15. Ibid., 84.

3 | THINK OF YOUR BOX AS AN HOURGLASS

WHILE EARLY PREVENTION IS A KEY FOR BUILD-ing a strong foundation going forward, where does that leave all of those who are past the adolescent stage? Is there any hope for reconnecting to that which was lost in the past? Absolutely, but the answer may reside in a place people would never think to look—an individual's habits.

Perhaps the word "habit" is overrated. The concept of building good habits is not a new one, but it is a highly prized concept in the world today. Many bestselling self-help books are founded on creating lives built around habits. Frank A. Clark once said, "A habit is something you can do without thinking—which is why most of us have so many of them."[1]

A habit implies a memorized pattern that never has to be thought about again. Phrases like "getting into the habit" and "making it a habit" are scattered throughout everyday conversation. But doesn't this defeat the purpose of mindful living? Instead, habits lead to mindless living. "To fall into a habit is to begin to cease to be."[2] Consider your drive to the grocery store. For many people, this drive has become so habitual that we often ask ourselves, "How did I get here, and what am I here for?" The brain gets so caught up in other thoughts and the drive to the store is such a habit that the person isn't even really present for the drive.

It is important to develop good and productive patterns. Individuals should work hard to make these patterns—which are mindfully incorporated at the appropriate time and place—a regular part of daily living. But life patterns don't have to be habits. Rather, they should reflect a natural part of the individual. For example, I would hope that we all want to be kind and loving. Is it better to be "naturally" kind and loving or "habitually" kind and loving? Is there a difference? Yes! It isn't *what* we do, but *why* we do it that counts. Habitually doing something implies that it can be done without thinking. This is called "unconsciousness," or acting without active awareness.

Naturally doing something, on the other hand, implies that the action is a part of the person. Naturally doing something includes being mindful and aware of the action. Ponder this question—if someone does something good solely out of habit, do they deserve the rewards for doing good when it was done so thoughtlessly?

Thoughtlessness is usually identified as a negative attribute, but isn't this how people live most of the time? Society has categorized, schedulized, and habitualized every moment, eliminating the need to think or even exist in the present. Life has become thoughtless in an effort to find time for life. Habit becomes a habit so much so that we praise the early adoption of habit and thoughtlessness.

It is often said that individuals should start early in their lives to make wise choices. If a choice is made early in life, it won't be necessary to make it again. The path to travel will have been selected. Consider the choice of whether or not to smoke. If someone makes the choice not to smoke while still young, he will never have to worry about being confronted with that choice again. Out of "habit," he will always choose not to smoke.

While choosing not to smoke is a good thing, it is also important to revisit why that choice was made earlier and *mindfully* reaffirm that choice each and every time the situation comes up. It is important to be within the moment; don't give away life through habit.

Habits actually lead to an unconscious acceptance of the mind–body–spirit disconnect. Over time, we develop the habit of ignoring our internal dialog. This could be called the "cookie" or "clean your room" syndrome. If a child wants a cookie or a parent wants a child to clean her room, they ask over and over again until the participants simply learn to ignore them. The longer the voice is ignored, the less it is actually heard. Soon, the requests are silenced due to lack of acknowledgement. The request may still be there, but the ability to listen has been lost.

This happens with our mind-body-spirit connection as well. There are those who have become so accomplished at ignoring what is going on inside that the signals no longer get through. It may be time to give up an attachment to the word "habit" in order to reconnect with the present.

This doesn't mean giving up the *process* of the habit—like taking a shower—it simply means completing the process mindfully. When was the last time someone paid attention to taking a shower? Does the exact same shower pattern happen almost daily? How about the pattern of brushing teeth? In general, if you were to start counting, you'd notice that you probably create the same brush strokes in the exact same pattern each time you brush your teeth.

It's interesting that most well-established habits tend to revolve around the physical body, so we give ourselves permission to "space out"—mentally going somewhere else while these tasks are completed. No wonder we have disconnected from our bodies. It's hard to even spend those few minutes of the day, which are exclusively set aside for the maintenance of the body, actually being present! Is it any surprise that our culture suffers from so much disease?

Think about the word "disease." Where did it originate? It is a combination of the word "dis," which is "to do the opposite of, deprive of, exclude, or expel from"; and "ease," which is "the state of being comfortable as freedom from pain, care, difficulty; naturalness."[3] Therefore, disease means to deprive of naturalness or exclude comfort.

People rarely start with a full-blown disease; they usually begin simply not feeling natural or comfortable. The problem is that the internal "nagging voice," which lets us know when something is wrong, has been turned off. The issue isn't recognized until it is screaming at us. Does this mean that all disease can be prevented or cured by being in touch with intuition and listening for dis-ease? No, but many instances of disease could be prevented from becoming extreme and debilitating if individuals simply paid more attention to the subtle feelings within the body. This lack of attention certainly sheds light upon the health of society today. The movement from dis-ease into disease is reflected in the ever-growing number of individuals suffering from chronic disease within our culture.

Chronic disease is commonly described as an ongoing condition that lasts more than three months.[4]

We recognize issues such as arthritis, obesity, diabetes, and so forth, as chronic diseases.

Today, chronic diseases, such as cardiovascular disease (primarily heart disease and stroke), cancer, and diabetes, are among the most prevalent, costly, and preventable of all health problems. Seven of every ten Americans who die each year (more than 1.7 million people) die of a chronic disease.[5]

Currently, obesity and type-2 diabetes are chronic diseases that are especially raging out of control. In 1990, the Center for Disease Control estimated that "no state had [obesity] prevalence equal to or greater than 15 percent. In 2007, only one state (Colorado) had prevalence less than 20 percent."[6] Statistics showing the prevalence rates of type-2 diabetes are similar. While type-2 diabetes is closely connected with an elderly population, the fastest growing diagnosed segment of our society is the age group 40 to 59 years of age.[7]

Interestingly, these are two areas that begin very commonly with dis-ease that goes unnoticed and unanswered. Obesity and type-2 diabetes may be directly linked to the habitual nature of daily action, which becomes unconscious and routine. Like the child asking for a cookie or the individual driving to the grocery store, many have "spaced out" and given up the connection to an internal dialog that would help them recognize symptoms and issues as they arise rather than waiting until they face a full-blown disease.

A disconcerting side effect of this internal disconnect is the conscious search for external answers about the body. Many are constantly looking and thinking "outside the box." This catchphrase has become a mantra for millions. It sounds so enlightened, so open-minded. Thinking outside the box seems to open up so many avenues for learning and improving lives through embracing external input.

What this phrase really implies is that somehow, a person is not enough as they are, or that a normal individual can't possibly have the right tools within to find answers—therefore, she must look to someone or something else for help. But when is the last time she actually looked *inside* her box? When is the last time she shook up the box? Chances are that all necessary answers will be found inside. Sometimes, a good internal shake-up is all it takes to reconnect.

Remember, the individual *is* the box. Everything within that box has created who we are today. What better foundation do we have on which to build who we will become tomorrow? We all can start thinking about the box as an hourglass; every once in a while, it needs to be shaken up and turned over to get the sand flowing again. The sand in the hourglass may never change, but each time it's shaken up, the placement and interaction of each grain of sand changes. It's a new configuration every time—always made from the original contents of the hourglass.

A great way to look at the contents of the individual box is to imagine building a house. If we only look at the contents of a toolbox, we will not see the finished house; rather, we'll see tools that can be mixed and matched in various circumstances in order to build the house.

Similarly, each box may not have all the answers to life's questions readily apparent in the box. But still, the tools will be there that we can mindfully mix and match to help make wise decisions and choices in any given situation. Does anyone have all the answers? Probably not, but hopefully one of the tools in the box is the wisdom to understand how to go about finding the answers that are right for the situation. Yoga may or may not be that tool. And that is all right. The best place to seek answers about health and disease control is internal. Think about it—only you can state definitively how it feels to be you. Only you can describe what is taking place inside, right this moment.

My students often ask how they should feel while doing a certain posture or breathing practice. I always reflect on the countless other aerobics and exercise classes I have attended over the years when a teacher would say, "Now you will feel this or that." "Wait," students would say. "What if I don't feel this or that? Am I doing it wrong?" This practice of second-guessing ourselves is instilled from an early age. We've all been taught cause and effect. Most of us were told what the answer should be in every circumstance and then were led to memorize that set of circumstances. We were taught to create habits of actions and outcomes.

The problems arise when the outcomes don't match the actions as expected. What causes this situation? Usually the culprit is something very simple—life. Consider this question: "Who said I should feel this way or that?" The answer is always the same: it's someone who felt a certain way when he was doing the task. It is important for us to remember we are not anyone else, so why should we expect to have the exact same experience? For that matter, each day is different, so why should we expect to have the same experience every day?

When students ask how they should feel in a pose, I respond, "This is what I feel, but you may feel something different. Why don't you listen a little closer to what's happening inside and then tell me what you experience in the pose." It's amazing how asking students to describe what is happening for them influences the entire class. Without fail, someone will mention an aspect of the pose that I haven't discussed. Then another student will speak up to confirm that she is experiencing what the first student described. It is powerful to share individual experience with others—not to convince them to feel the same, but to give others permission to recognize alternatives that might not have been expressed by the teacher. This is a true teaching moment—when learning occurs as a group. This is the essence of experiential therapy.

When you honor who you are today and recognize your own intuition, you begin to think from the inside out. Instead of listening to what someone else professes is the right answer for how to exercise, what to eat, or how to be healthy, you begin to intuitively recognize what works for you. Remember, who said everyone should be a size 2? Someone who's a size 2! Who said we all should be able to touch our toes? Someone who can touch her toes! Who said we should eat only certain foods? Someone who does! Get the picture?

Experts invite people to think outside the box. What they really mean is, "Come inside MY box—it's better than yours." They tell us to give up our individual ways of living and adopt their approach to success by creating habits as they have. The media tells of someone who has had great results losing weight or gaining strength by doing "Exercise X" or "Diet Y," so everyone blindly adopts these ideas through a "one-size-fits-all" mentality. If it worked for one person, it must surely work for everyone.

Yoga teaches students to be present, to listen to the subtle, and to connect or reconnect with the whole being. Yoga teaches students how to be their best selves. Being your best self is a common catch-phrase in current culture. The problem is that most of us have bought into the idea that our best self should to be the same as everyone else. We should be thin, be fit, be blonde, be young, be popular. We should have flawless skin, great teeth, a successful career, a happy family. All these things may be true—for somebody. But, just because it's true doesn't make it relevant.

There is only so much space in each day and only so much energy in each individual. Mindfulness is so important because it teaches students to intuitively connect inside and recognize what they have space for in their unique and individual lives. People always expect that they will get better every day at certain tasks, yet yoga teaches that students shouldn't expect to be better at things today than they were yesterday because they are different each day. What if tomorrow a student is sick or has an accident and loses some ability? Does this mean that life is over because he can't be better at things today than he was yesterday? No! The only thing to become better at is listening to each day and recognizing what it can bring.

Many students have a hard time letting go of certain habits when they practice balancing poses. It helps to remind them that their bodies are different every day and that balancing is one of the most challenging things to approach mindfully. We feel like it should happen the same way every time. Students eventually recognize that their bodies are mostly made of water and that their water levels fluctuate daily.

Imagine carrying a pan of water to the stove. You consciously consider the size of the pan and the amount of water inside. Then you reflect back to past experience to confirm how much effort this task will take. Yet, even with all of your preparation and past experience with this situation, you still need to be mindfully aware of carrying the pan without spilling any of the water. It is a true balancing act! You can't simply move the pan out of habit because the situation is always a little bit different from the last time you did it. You must listen to the combination of the circumstances today to be able to successfully complete the task.

Consider the weight lifting competition in the Olympics. The athletes put chalk on their hands; they approach the weight bar; they squat and wrap their hands around the bar and connect with the task. Many times, they will let go of the bar and then regrasp it before lifting. What changes? The bar doesn't change, their hands don't change, the chalk may change slightly—if they put more on or wipe some off—but the elements of the activity don't really change. What changes is the connection of all the elements within that moment—the "aha" instant when everything feels right. Now the lift can happen.

This is how to become the best self. When we truly connect with the intuitive subtle voice within and "zip together our ski coats," the desire to conform will melt away, and the awareness of our individual fabulous beings will emerge.

So, how do you start the process of looking inside your own box? How do you shake yourself up? Simply open the dialog to discover what is there. As I was finishing a yoga class at CFC one evening, I instructed the students to lie on their backs in a relaxed manner and begin breathing. I encouraged them to let go of stress and tension through breathing deeply.

One student said that she didn't know how to let go of tension, and she couldn't figure out how to relax. I thought for a moment. Then I asked her if she had told herself to let go. She looked at me as if she didn't understand, and I asked her if she had tried actually saying the words in her mind, "Let go of tension in my neck." Had she consciously told her body what she expected of it? Her reply was, "Of course not." The thought had never even crossed her mind. Who ever heard of talking to yourself and telling yourself what to do?

Don't we convey this idea to one other in an off-handed sort of way? When we know someone who is nervous or anxious, we try to help by saying, "Just breathe and relax."

Sometimes, you may tell yourself to "just relax." But this is merely a vague idea. The important thing is to have a meaningful dialog, not just a random and generalized thought. Be specific and address the issue. Don't just tell yourself to relax; tell yourself to relax your toes or shoulders. Don't just tell yourself to breathe; tell yourself to breathe into the place where you are holding tension. You must tell yourself what you want and expect. Gain control of your internal voice.

Many people create lists and plans and goals all the time. We've all been taught that if we verbalize and write something down, we will be more successful. Brian Kim, an expert in self-improvement, has stated, "I'm sure you've heard this advice before. Write your goals down. If they're not written down, they're just dreams. When you write things down, it sets off a chain of events that will change your life. I am a firm believer of writing."[8] Verbalizing goals is as essential as writing them down.

This may sound silly, and you may doubt the success of simply talking to yourself, but give it a try. Take a moment to look inside the box and see what is going on. "Speak to the unspoken."[9]

NOTES

1. "Frank A. Clark Quotes," accessed March 5, 2009, http://thinkexist.com/quotes/frank_a._clark/3.html.
2. Miguel de Unamuno, *The Tragic Sense of Life* (New York: Dover Publications, 1954), 124.
3. *Merriam-Webster Online,* s.v. "disease," accessed March 2, 2009, http://www.merriam-webster.com/dictionary.

4. "Chronic Diseases and Health Promotion," Centers for Disease Control and Prevention, http://www.cdc.gov/nccdphp.

5. Ibid.

6. "U.S. Obesity Trends," Centers for Disease Control and Prevention, http://www.cdc.gov/nccdphp/dnpa/obesity/trend/maps/obesity_trends_2007.pdf.

7. "National Diabetes Statistics," NDIC, accessed March 4, 2009, http://diabetes.niddk.nih.gov/DM/PUBS/statistics.

8. Brian Kim, "Why You Should Write Down Your Goals," *The Definitive Guide to Self Improvement* (blog), August 1, 2006, http://briankim.net/blog/2006/08/why-you-should-write-down-your-goals.

9. "About YogaMotion," Nancy Ruby's YogaMotion, accessed March 1, 2009, http://www.yogamotion.com/about_yogamotion.html.

4 | SHIFT HAPPENS!

I WANT TO CHANGE! PEOPLE SAY THIS ALL THE time. What is change? How does it happen? Does it "stick?" Usually not. A perfect example of the inability to truly change can be found in the diet and weight loss industry. Why is this industry booming? Because it continues to create life-long customers based on the principle that change doesn't last.

The weight regain rate has been estimated at 90 percent.[1] No wonder there are so many diet and weight loss products. Society is addicted to external answers that promise to help create change; however, the change doesn't last, so people have to continue to buy new products. The fitness industry has mystified the process of staying healthy and created a dependence on expert advice that changes every year. One year, we are directed to do isolation muscle work, and the next year we are told to do massive amounts of cardio exercise.

In her book, *The Fitness Instinct*, Peg Jordan discusses how far away individuals have moved from their intuitive selves by embracing the expertise of the "health industry," all in the effort to conform to what is expected. "Making it harder than it is—that's how any profession robs you of your own intuitive know-how. . . . The fitness profession is no different. . . . We must now rely on scientists and experts, instead of our own common sense, to figure out how to be fit."[2]

The "experts" within the diet and fitness industry lead us to believe that we are unable to understand what is right for us, so we must rely on them for correct answers.

The only permanent change is the creation of our dependence on their advice. Somewhere along the way, "exercise science mastery became the exclusive domain of specialists who had achieved advanced levels of education and experience."[3] This emphasis on science and exercise became prevalent in the 1980s with the increased emphasis on heart disease research and prevention. Although the government spent massive amounts of time and energy on protocols to help people change their behavior, many individuals were still suffering.

"It was only when we had many individuals who were still having heart attacks despite doing everything we recommended that we began to question what other biological, emotional, psychological, and genetic factors might be at work."[4] Science may not have all the answers, but society still places extreme trust in these "experts." We rely on instruction from others because we're told that we can't be objective about ourselves. But this reliance on external answers does not improve objectivity; rather, it breeds contempt.

Just walk into any local gym, and it won't be long until you hear the biases of the so-called "experts." Conversation quickly moves to the "guilt" stage, with the personal trainer or teacher telling the students that they are lazy, that they don't want to change badly enough, that they are making excuses not to work hard, and that they just need to push through. Jordan states, "I believe unconscionable reactions such as this reflect an arrogance and steel-edged superiority that are fostered by the strength-training and body-shaping cults of the fitness movement. Their script goes like this: 'I know what's better for you than you do . . . so just pay up and shut up.' "[5]

I was very sick one week, so I had to stay in bed most of the time. After watching TV for a while, I realized that advertising for diet and weight loss is everywhere. In an hour's time during the middle of the day, I counted five advertisements for supplements, equipment, and eating plans targeted at this issue. These advertisements were on the same channel in a single hour! What does this teach adults? What does this teach children? These products are so prevalent because so many fall back into original habits. Change is hard—it usually doesn't last. The diet and fitness industry depends on this.

Who is to blame? In the United States alone, $40 billion per year is spent on diet products.[6] Someone out there is making a *lot* of money! But someone out there is also *spending* a lot of money! We're facing the age-old paradox: which came first, the chicken or the egg? It would be easy to blame everything on the diet and fitness industry for creating such a problem; yet the problem would not exist—at least not to the extent it does—if the population didn't demand such quick-fix answers. On the other hand, people wouldn't crave this type of change if they weren't bombarded constantly with the idea that they must be thinner, stronger, and supposedly healthier.

According to the FDA, approximately 8 million Americans will begin some type of controlled weight-loss program each year. These programs include liquid diets, controlled and portioned meals, and medically monitored regimens.[7] This number does not include the millions who will buy into fad and over-the-counter (OTC) diet supplements that aren't monitored in a controlled environment. In a 2002 report specifically addressing weight-loss advertising, the Federal Trade Commission (FTC) reported that "at any given time, 70 million Americans are trying to lose weight or prevent weight gain."[8]

While many physicians recommend a 5 to 15 percent weight-loss goal for the majority of patients, "[t]he public often perceives weight losses of 5 to 15 percent as small and insufficient, even though they suffice to prevent and improve many of the problems associated with weight gain, overeating, and a sedentary life style."[9] Why do people feel this way? Because they are inundated with visual testimonials of extreme weight loss.

Diet and weight-loss advertising has moved from general comments about losing weight into the arena of personal testimonials. The media touts "before and after" photos to supposedly "prove" that extreme changes in body composition are now possible without any effort! During a follow up report in 2004, the FTC noted a distinct increase and change in weight-loss advertising.

FTC staff compared weight-loss product advertising that appeared in 1992 in the February through May issues of eight national magazines (Cosmopolitan, Family Circle, Glamour, Ladies Home Journal, McCall's/Rosie, Redbook, Self, and Woman's Day) with advertising that appeared in the same magazines in 2001. Between 1992 and 2001, the number of weight-loss products advertised in these magazines more than doubled, and the number of distinct advertisements for those products more than tripled.

Between 1992 and 2001, the types of products advertised also shifted, from primarily meal replacements such as diet shakes to primarily dietary supplements.[10]

This increased volume of advertising, along with the new emphasis on taking a pill rather than replacing a meal, has created an environment of "diet mania" that is difficult to escape. It is especially interesting to note the change from meal replacement shakes, which would typically eliminate a high-calorie meal, toward dietary supplements, which claim that no change in eating habits is necessary. It's easy to see why this change took place. If we don't actually have to *do* anything to change except take a pill, we might be tempted to try that change!

Another new trend of highly persuasive advertising is the "before and after" testimonials. When presented with a photo of someone who looks run-down and out of shape before she took the "magic potion," only to be miraculously transformed into a happy and active swimsuit model after taking the advertised supplement, who wouldn't want to buy into the dream? But the majority of these claims are unrealistic, if not impossible. Think Photoshop. "The world of weight-loss advertising is a virtual fantasy land where pounds 'melt away' while 'you continue to eat your favorite foods': 'amazing pills . . . seek and destroy enemy fat.' It's a world where, in spite of prevailing scientific opinion, no sacrifice is required to lose weight."[11]

So, who is trustworthy? These two reports created by the FTC offer great insights into the world of diet and weight-loss marketing. They open our eyes to the reality that diet and weight-loss advertising is a multi-billion-dollar industry that isn't likely to be looking out for its customers' best interests. The FTC reports list numerous "red flags" to watch for and identify the claims of many over-the-counter diet supplements as being misleading, if not outright untruthful and fraudulent.[12]

On her website, Junkfood Science, Sandy Szwarc posted a special report containing additional information regarding the FTC research project. Her article, entitled "Junkfood Science Special Report: FTC's diet pill crackdown—a marketing scheme in disguise" (2007), notes: "On January 4, the Federal Trade Commission announced it had cracked down on makers of four over-the-counter (OTC) weight-loss pills for making false advertising claims, fining them $25 million."[13] This sounds great on the surface, doesn't it?

What is not fully examined within the FTC research, though, are the formally controlled diet programs. These are typically programs based on membership and/or purchase of portioned meals and supplements. Also excluded from the report were any references to surgical options such as gastric bypass. Why weren't these included in the report? Ironically, many corporate leaders of formal weight-loss programs and physician coalitions just so happened to be members of the "professional" board that helped to write the FTC report. Szwarc offers her opinion on this missing piece of the weight-loss and diet crazed industry. "By crippling a significant hunk of their competition—OTC weight-loss products, which now rake in $1 billion a year—more consumers will be led to their products. They are not passive beneficiaries of these FTC actions. For years they have actively participated in an extensive, well-planned marketing strategy."[14]

Szwarc identifies key leaders from the American Society of Bariatric Physicians (gastric bypass and other surgeries), the American Obesity Association (a lobbying group funded largely by pharmaceutical companies), Jenny Craig, Inc., Slimfast Foods Company, and Weight Watchers International, Inc., as well as many others, as members of the partnership that made up the coalition spearheaded by the FTC to research and generate their report.

She notes that the introduction of the 2002 FTC report "was written by George Blackburn, past president of NAASO, Board member of the American Obesity Association, and a trustee of the Slimfast Nutritional Institute."[15] According to Szwarc, the majority of the forty-one coalition members who participated in drafting the report had a conflict of interest issue due to their financial involvement with specific weight-loss industries and entities, which conveniently, are not targeted within the study. Obviously, the coalition was only interested in removing their competition and not in diminishing the diet and weight-loss industry. Does this mean that all weight-loss advocates are enemies? Not necessarily. However, it means that we should be actively questioning why they do what they do.

How can the cycle be broken? What can truly change? We can't simply tell the industry to not advertise. We can only create change within ourselves. If we give up our own voices, we give power to the external voices clamoring for influence. Then we blame these voices for speaking, pushing our personal responsibility onto the shoulders of anyone who will give us the answer we want to hear. When we don't get the desired results from a pill or a product, we backslide into recidivism, which is what the diet and fitness industry is counting on. People change; then they change right back!

I'm fascinated by the word "recidivism." It means "a tendency to relapse into a previous condition or mode of behavior."[16] Society usually associates this word with criminals who repeatedly commit the same crimes. But recidivism can just as easily apply to any aspect of life—most notably New Year's resolutions.

Have you ever made a New Year's resolution you didn't keep? Do you make the same resolutions every year? What prevents you from following through? Why don't you change? Because change is really hard to hold on to. But shift happens!

Here's an example I use with my students: Stand up and look directly forward. Pay attention to all that you can see, especially in the periphery of your vision. Now close your eyes and turn the opposite direction. Open your eyes and look directly forward. What do you see? Is there anything that is the same in the two views, even in the periphery? Probably not much, if anything.

This is change. When we turn 180 degrees, we give up the entirety of the first view to get a new view. We lose everything we had at first and replace it with something else. Typically, this is what change requires. It asks us to totally give up one thing and to replace it with something else. When life is easy (notice the use of "ease") and uncomplicated, we can deal with this change for a while. As soon as life gets uneasy (similar to "dis-ease"), we retreat to that which is familiar and known. Almost everyone will seek that which is comfortable, easy, and thoughtless. They go back to habits.

So, I ask my students to stand and look directly forward, paying special attention to what they see in the periphery. Next, I ask them to turn slightly to the left and look straight ahead. Notice that some of what they were able to see in their right periphery is gone, but they have gained something in their left periphery. Additionally, what was previously in the left periphery is now moving closer to center. They are giving up a little of what was not really central to their gaze and gently bringing something else into better focus. They are changing the center of their gaze and redefining what they see. Slowly, I move the students a few inches at a time until they have turned 180 degrees. They have changed their focus because SHIFT HAPPENS!

Shift begins in the mind—in beliefs and attitudes. Do we ever ask ourselves, "Where did I get this idea or that belief?" Many beliefs and attitudes have been formed by peer pressure or what is considered the social norm—because everyone is doing it. Adults often counsel youth to not give into peer pressure and to think for themselves. Yet as adults, we give in to peer pressure every day. Oh, we don't recognize it as peer pressure; rather, we mistake peer pressure for fact-based truth.

The diet and fitness industry is inundated with concepts that started as someone's opinion but through the years have been adopted as necessary for good health and longevity. For example, the health industry may argue that the astronomical increases in human longevity result from new adaptations of exercise and diet. In reality, increased life span is more closely related to the advent of cleaner drinking water and advancements in sanitation; yes, plumbers are to thank for long life! Yet, it would be hard to convince people to question the current approaches to diet and exercise. Once an idea is embraced and placed in the mainstream, it is extremely difficult to change. Health and wellness ideas are also often overused. People tend to embrace the idea that if a little is good, a lot must be better.

Different personalities will reflect philosophy in different ways, yet eventually, we all seem to fall into the same patterns. When presented with fresh information, we tend to use this newfound knowledge to approach every aspect of our lives. We have forgotten how to be mindful and consider different approaches for different situations. We embrace the concept of change and decide to paint our entire existence with this new brush. We have forgotten how to simply shift—not change. Even when we shift instead of change, some of us may choose to shift back, but we do it with mindfulness and respect for the moment.

I am always reminded of this principle when I encounter students with an extensive background in other forms of activity. During one of my community yoga classes, a student was very upset that I was teaching students to inhale and exhale through the nose. After class, she stated that she was a voice coach and was not following the breathing techniques she ing her vocal lessons. I carefully considered her concern and reminded her that just because we use certain techniques with certain tasks doesn't mean that we should always use these techniques.

When we practice various breathing exercises in yoga class, I guide the students to breathe in and out through the nose for some techniques and to utilize other breathing styles for other techniques. One technique even requires alternate nostril breathing—but I wouldn't recommend it for every moment of the day! I reminded her that she was still free to use different breathing techniques for singing, but isn't it nice to expand our hourglass to find other techniques we might want to incorporate into our lives?

Options and multiple approaches—when introduced and embraced mindfully—can be very life affirming, especially when old habits can't support new situations. Sometimes we get so caught up in new experiences and new ideas that we overflow life with them or reject them out of hand because they oppose previous knowledge.

This issue also comes up often with many dancers who practice yoga. Without fail, every class I teach includes someone with a dancing background who struggles with the physical differences between how they have been trained to move in dance and how yoga asks them to move. I listen carefully to their concerns and then encourage the students to recognize that I am not asking them to give up their dancing techniques—

just like I didn't ask the singer to give up her breathing technique. I'm merely asking my students to put those techniques aside and mindfully move within the framework of yoga technique for this class only. Just as I would never tell a dancer to use yoga techniques in ballet class if it was in opposition to what she was trying to accomplish, I help her recognize the trouble with using certain ballet techniques in yoga class. Many things in yoga and dance are similar, but many movements are in direct opposition to each other, and it requires mindfulness and a willingness to truly be present in order to move away from habit and into the practice of the moment.

So, why is shift so important? Unlike change, shift only asks that you move at your own pace toward goals. Shift allows for time and reflection, for questioning and confirming. When you mindfully incorporate the principle of shift rather than change, you allow for an internal dialog to dictate whether or not you end up changed. Is a certain exercise or diet right for you? The initial answer should *never* be a "yes" or "no." It should *always* be "maybe." The final answer will come after you begin shifting into the process and exploring the journey.

Sometimes it's hard to allow shift to happen because we are accustomed to the uncomfortable demands of change; we might worry that shift has the same demands. But if we keep in mind that we will only shift what we are ready to give up and are only introducing a small amount of newness to life at a time, our perceptions will flow together. Soon we won't even remember what we shifted away from and what we shifted toward. We may even find that the shift was a temporary necessity or that the shift was a needful new focus for permanence.

When shift is allowed to happen, it will feel natural not forced. When shift is allowed to happen, it will enhance life without depleting it. When shift is allowed to happen, it will be a movement toward the true self.

NOTES

1. Diane Woznicki, "The Ups and Downs of Weight-Loss Programs," *Priorities for Health* 3, no. 4 (Fall 1991): 23.

2. Peg Jordan, *The Fitness Instinct: the Revolutionary New Approach to Healthy Exercise that Is Fun, Natural, and No Sweat* (Pennsylvania: Rodale Press, 1999), 3.

3. Ibid., 6.

4. Ibid., 7.

5. Ibid., 9.

6. "The Diet Industry: A Big Fat Lie," BusinessWeek Debate Room, accessed March 10, 2009, http://www. businessweek.com/debateroom/archives/2008/01/the_ diet_ indust.html.

7. "The Facts About Weight Loss Products and Programs," Food and Drug Administration, last modified September 3, 1993, accessed April 30, 2009, http://www.cfsan.fda. gov/~dms/wgtloss.html.

8. "Weight-Loss Advertising: An Analysis of Current Trends,"

Federal Trade Commission Staff Report, September 2002, http://www.ftc.gov/bcp/reports /weightloss.pdf.

9. Ibid.

10. "2004 Weight-Loss Advertising Survey," Federal Trade Commission Staff Report, April 2005, http://www2.ftc.gov/os/2005/04/050411weightlosssurvey 04.pdf.

11. Weight-loss Advertising Analysis, 18.

12. Ibid., 6.

13. Sandy Szwarc, "Junkfood Science Special Report: FTC's Diet Pill Crackdown—a Marketing Scheme in Disguise," *Junkfood Science* (blog), January 8, 2007, http://junkfoodscience.blogspot.com/2007/01/junkfood-science-special-report-ftcs.html.

14. Ibid.

15. Ibid.

16. *Merriam-Webster Online*, s.v. "recidivism," accessed March 2, 2009, http://www.merriam-webster.com/dictionary.

5 | SO, WHAT'S EATING YOU?

STUDENTS OFTEN ASK ME, "HOW CAN I GET MY kids to eat healthier foods?" This question always makes my toes curl because I know what comes next. The rest of the story goes something like this: "I don't allow junk food into my house, and I constantly tell them not to eat this or that because it is bad for them, but they eat it at school or their friend's house anyway. What can I do? I am trying to teach them to eat good things and to exercise because I don't want them to get fat, but it doesn't seem to change their behavior."

There is that word again—change. My initial reply always earns a raised eyebrow and a puzzled look: "The first problem is that we identify food as good and bad," I say. Well, that is the last thing my students expect to hear! Can't I just give them the words to say to make their kids do what they want?

Our culture has created a phenomenon known

as disordered eating. This is not necessarily the same as having an eating disorder; rather, it is a distorted relationship with food. There are many reasons for disordered eating. A simple one has come from our ancestors—all with good intentions. Did your parents or grandparents ever issue the order to clean your plate before they would serve dessert? There is nothing wrong with this sentiment. Remember, there are starving children all over the world (how many times has this been said?).

Statements like these instill within us a judgment about types of food: dinner food is to be endured while desserts are a prize! We eat everything on our plates regardless of our fullness and then still find room for dessert because we've earned it! In the next breath, society says not to eat too many desserts and treats because they are bad for our health. How can we reconcile these two ideas? What does this teach kids? No wonder they are confused—so are adults! In the effort to be good parents, we look to "experts" for answers. It's difficult to instill a healthy attitude toward food within our children when we don't have one ourselves.

Another question that my students ask is, "How can I get my kids to not want to eat as soon as they get home from school? It ruins their dinner." I like to turn the question around and ask, "Are the kids ruining their dinner or are they ruining your dinner?"

Then I engage in a conversation to get the students thinking about what goals they have for having family dinner. Is family dinner a time to make sure your children are fed and satisfied, or is it really about bringing the family together? If it's the former, then let the kids eat when they are hungry. If it's the latter, then let them eat when they are hungry after school but require them to sit and interact with the family at the table during dinner.

An interesting thing usually happens when my students try this approach. The kids are uncomfortable just sitting and watching everyone else eat. They pay more attention to their hunger cues after school and recognize that maybe they just need something to hold them over until dinnertime instead of a big snack. I can't claim this works every time, but it is a really good starting point for teaching the process of intuitive eating to our children. It also helps us, as parents, be more mindful about our own relationship with food. How do you feel about food?

This is a quiz I give my students. Be honest when considering your answers.

1. Have you ever stated that you won't eat a certain food because it's bad for you?
2. Have you ever restricted more than one food group, perhaps refined sugar and excessive dairy products, red meats, or excessive starches or carbohydrates?

3. Have you ever agreed with the idea that you shouldn't eat anything after a certain time of day?

4. Have you ever decided that the restriction or elimination of certain foods from your diet must be healthy and good?

5. Have you ever said, "I just want to lose five pounds so I can fit into my dress this weekend, so I'll only eat once a day for the next 6 days"?

6. After a large holiday meal, such as Thanksgiving dinner, have you ever jokingly said, "I am so full I should just throw up, and then I'll feel better"?

Do you recognize yourself in any of these situations? If so, you may be among the millions of people practicing disordered eating. Disordered eating is not only about the actual consumption of food; it also encompasses thoughts about food and discussions of food—or food talk.

We use food talk unconsciously and out of habit. We say things like, "If you eat that, it will go right to your hips." Or, "I can't believe I ate the whole thing." Or, "I'll have to do an extra twenty minutes on the treadmill to make up for this." Or, "I know I shouldn't eat this, but I'll be good later," and so forth.

We speak this way because we have been conditioned over the past few decades to equate food consumption directly with the pursuit of health—or at the very least, the pursuit of thinness. We judge our own value and the value of others by using food consumption as an outward marker of self control, which results in habitual negative conversations about food.

We don't even have to know the person we are judging—we merely attribute words such as "weak-willed" and "unhealthy" to complete strangers as we project our own distorted relationship with food onto others. Society has given a moral value to food that allows for a moral judgment of people. Is there ever a positive conversation about food? Does anyone ever discuss enjoyment of food without feeling guilty? Are we falling ever deeper into the trap of food talk? How did food become so powerful?

Most of us have done this at one time or another. But if we feel such a desire to change, we need to ask ourselves some very honest questions: "Why do I feel the need to change my eating habits? If I wouldn't gain or lose weight from either eating what I was told to eat or eating what I wanted to eat, which would I choose? Is it really about eating so-called healthier foods or about losing weight?" Be honest!

Why does everyone want to lose weight? The desire to be thin is a fairly new concept within the course of history. Less than a hundred years ago, the pinnacle of beauty was to display excess body fat. Being too thin was seen as a sign of poor health and living standards. Fatness was a sign of success and beauty. Popular magazines of the day even wrote articles containing tips on how to put on those extra pounds. One such article was published by Ritter & Co. in 1891. In the advertisement, the company states:

> Respectfully tell the ladies to GET PLUMP with Professor Williams' famed 'Fat-Ten-U' Foods. Why suffer tortures with inferior mechanical devices that artificially fatten? Don't look like the poor unfortunate . . . who, shorn of her artificial inflationary devices & pads, must, in the confines of her bedroom, through shame, try to cover her poor thin figure from the gaze of her beloved spouse.[1]

Think about it! Just a century ago, it was considered shameful to be thin and without a womanly figure. What has changed? Nothing, really. The emphasis has merely moved from one extreme to the other. We are still listening to the "experts" who tell us we are somehow lacking. The question is no longer *what* we do, but *why* we do it What is the motivation to eat what is "good" for us?

At the Center for Change, we practice intuitive eating. "Since first teaching its concepts in 1999, the Center for Change has been a pioneer in using the concept of "intuitive eating."[2]

Registered and clinical dietician Kim Passmore reflects the need to create a renewed relationship with food. "Intuitive eating not only helps individuals get back in touch with their body's internal cues, it also helps them to stop their battle against food and learn how to "make peace" with it."[3]

Rebekah Hennes, a pioneer in the use of intuitive eating for eating disorders, states, "Food is just food. There is no good or bad food. Every food is okay and nourishing in some aspect. After food is broken down, the body doesn't know where the protein, carbohydrate, or fat came from. It cannot tell if the carbohydrate, fat, protein mix came from a cookie and milk or salad with meat and cheese. However, the body needs a mix of these three fuels in order to function well."[4]

Again, it is important to honestly consider the question, "Why do we feel the need to eat 'good' foods, and why do we classify other foods as bad?" Perhaps, as adults, we should just do what children do—we should eat when we're hungry and stop when we're full. We should listen to what we feel like eating.

It's true: there *are* some children who will never actually understand or feel that they have to eat, but these cases are extremely rare. Regardless, this concept still holds valid—all we need to do is listen to our bodies in order to recognize when we're satisfied. It seems easy, but it's not. We don't normally trust ourselves to just stop eating cookies, right? Well, have you ever had to eat only cookies for a whole day because there was nothing else? Did you ever want to eat a cookie again?

Most people initially believe that by using internal cues to guide food amounts and food choices, they will inevitably be "unhealthy," make the wrong choices, and eat too much. This is a sign of a lack of self-trust, which is natural when external factors have been used for so long to make these choices for us. Regaining trust is a process. It takes time and practice, but it is well worth it.[5]

Most of our desires and cravings stem from a restriction someone has placed on food. A key element of intuitive eating is to stay present and to truly experience food. Does our society encourage enjoying a meal or merely eating? Do we put food into our mouths as an unconscious robotic movement while doing something else—like watching TV or driving?

Unlike merely taking in food, intuitively eating a meal requires presence of mind and engagement of all the senses. It requires something really scary—we must actually stay present and feel what is going on inside as we take care of our bodies. When this happens, we become intuitive about the process. Intuitive eating is hard! Learning to trust the self again is overwhelming, especially after years of listening to everyone else's directions. The important thing to remember is that honesty is an important part of rebuilding this trust.

Do most people identify *craving* with sweets or "junk" food? This really isn't intuitive—it's habitual. If we're truly honest with ourselves and we take a moment to listen to what our bodies are really craving, we will intuitively moderate and balance our diet. It's like magic—but it takes a lot of work, trust, and honesty! Rebekah Hennes offers a few tips for incorporating and embracing intuitive eating successfully:

1. No scales, measuring tapes, measuring spoons, or cups.
2. No label reading, counting calories, or planning menus.
3. Never diet again.
4. Do not label foods as good or bad.
5. Participate only in forms of exercise that you enjoy and that help you to feel good.
6. Eat what you like and savor the eating experience. Taste your food, relax, and check out the taste in the middle of the meal. Does it still taste good? If it doesn't taste good, don't eat it. If you love it, savor it.
7. Eat at least three meals a day.
8. Regarding food: be more cautious about under-doing it than over-doing it. Over-doing it evens out more easily in the long run. Under-doing it sets you up for the restrict-binge-purge cycle.[6]

Learning to eat intuitively takes a lot of faith and practice. It is not a quick fix or magic pill. It is a long-term approach that is definitely worth all the hard work put into it.

In addition to food issues, my students often ask

me other health questions. Runners want to know why they aren't able to stretch as much as other students in class and how to overcome this. They want to gain flexibility without losing their running capacity. I try to explain that they have created a runner's body, so there are limitations to what they may want to introduce in the form of flexibility. It is a trade-off, but so is everything else in life. We just don't want to acknowledge this because society tells us that we can have it all. This is the power of choice—deciding which trade-off is most beneficial.

For runners, the muscles in their legs have been trained to satisfy the demands of running, and if they become more flexible, they will see a change in their ability to run. At first, they don't care. They just want to be like everyone else in class. Predictably, this attitude of comparison with others leads to an internal conflict and an opportunity to really be honest with themselves.

One student was concerned because the stretching felt really good, but his running times were slowing down. I suggested that he not try to stretch so deeply in class because he needed those muscles to work in a different way for running.

After a few months, he told me that he wasn't ready to give up running, so he had decided that yoga wasn't right for him. He didn't want to feel like a beginner in class and was unwilling to stay on a moderate level during the practice, so he chose to stick with running for the present.

Another student, however, had the opposite experience. When she first started coming to class, she was an avid runner and had extremely tight hamstrings. She was frustrated in class because of her lack of flexibility and wanted to improve this area. I asked her about running and found out that it was one of the most important things in her life. She loved running! She enjoyed the outdoors and the feeling of "going." I gave her my standard "runner's disclaimer" about working moderately with stretches during yoga class so that her running wouldn't be too negatively impacted. She agreed to modify her expectations of flexibility.

We worked for a few weeks and spoke often after class about the concept of really being present during activity and feeling what is happening to our bodies as we engage in movement. She became very expressive about the new sensations she was discovering through yoga practice and how this made her feel even more alive within her own body.

One day after class, she told me she wasn't enjoying running as much because she was now more aware of her body and how it felt to run. She recognized the strain on her ankles and knees and didn't like the feeling. I reminded her of her beginning days of yoga when she wasn't sure if yoga was for her.

At that time, she had insisted that running was her

life and she loved it. Now, however, she was mindful of a movement away from her long-held desire to constantly run and was embracing her newfound enjoyment of all different types of movement. We talked about how shift happens. And it was certainly happening to her. An interesting side effect of this shift was her redefined connection to "going." She had always associated running with truly feeling alive and active; now she was recognizing that it didn't take fast-paced movement to create this sensation, it merely required attention and complete immersion in the moment.

I am constantly reminding students that life is about choices and turns in the road. We can't travel all roads at the same time. We have to make choices about which road we want to be on right now. The hard thing to recognize is that every time we consciously choose one road, we give up—for a time—the possible destinations of other roads.

This truth is brought to the forefront in yoga. While each student brings a different history with him, yoga practice requires students to make choices that may move away from earlier experiences. They must give up one thing to make room for something else. They must choose whether this is the right time to allow shift to happen or if, like my former student, they are content with their current path and not ready to make the shift that yoga requires. There's no right or wrong answer—unless we make harmful choices—but we each need to recognize and mindfully acknowledge that not all things are possible at the same time. We also need to recognize that time exists. We aren't today who we were yesterday or ten years ago. We need to embrace who we are today, but sometimes this can be hard to do.

Over the years, I have worked with many students who have had difficulty accepting this concept. Our conversations sound something like this: "I used to be a [dancer/athlete/other], and I used to be able to do this with ease. I am out of shape right now, but my goal is to get back to where I was when I was twenty."

I had an interesting ongoing conversation with one student, who was really struggling with being at a different place now, in her late forties, than she had been in her twenties. She felt as if life was pretty much meaningless unless she could recapture the fabulous life, as she perceived it, from her earlier years. I asked her if she would be willing to give up her husband, children, and grandchildren to go back to that time.

She had to really think about her answer and was even willing to give up some of her current life to recapture what she considered were her best years. Although we spoke several times on this subject, my student was still convinced that nothing in her current or future life could ever be as wonderful as her past experiences.

I teach my students that we are never the same from one day to the next. How can we be? Through the lifecycle, our body entirely replaces almost every cell in approximately seven years; so, about every seven years, we are completely new people. The cells we have today aren't the same ones that did the splits when we were teenagers. We can never be the same person we were when we were twenty. I don't think I would even *want* to be! But that's beside the point.

The important issue is to recognize that every moment is a new and exciting experience. Living in the past and defining ourselves by what we used to be or do merely brings discouragement to the present. If we are truly living mindfully, we will honor each moment as the most important of our lives. This moment is the only one in which we are alive.

While we may not be able to recapture our youth, we can definitely work on bringing new and improved energy to our present life. A few years ago, I worked with a student who was having trouble with her feet. For years, she had gone to orthopedic doctors because her arches bothered her so much. She was continually getting new and stronger inserts for her shoes. She had been diagnosed with "hammer toe," and the doctor wanted her to use a new insert with a cutout below the ball of her foot where the hammer toe was pushing. The idea was to make room, allowing the bulging hammer toe to relax.

She had been coming to yoga class for about a year. She said that every time she got new inserts, her feet would hurt even worse after class. I wasn't a doctor, but I did have a background in anatomy and physiology, so I offered to work with her to see if we could alleviate some of her pain.

I explained that while I personally believed inserts for shoes were beneficial to many people with arch problems, I felt that too often people relied on the build of their shoe to compensate for the lack of strength in the foot muscles. It is much easier to cure than to prevent. It is much easier to get an insert to do the work that our feet should be doing.

I asked if she would be willing to try going without shoes for an hour every day and simply walking around her house or yard. I gave her some exercises to practice while she was doing this, like lifting her toes while she stood in place, making sure that she stood with her feet in a neutral position and hip-width apart, and so forth.

I encouraged her to massage her feet and feel what was going on with the bones and muscles. I also encouraged her to be more aware of the way she placed energy into her feet when standing and to try to create a more balanced condition by placing weight into the ball mount of her big toe and her pinky toe and the inside and outside point of her heel, and to concentrate energy along the outside edge of her foot while engaging the muscles of her arch.

After a few months, she reported that pain from her hammer toe had lessened. She was occasionally even going entire days without wearing her inserts. Now, I don't claim that yoga cured her or that I am in any way a doctor. I simply reminded her that people have been without shoes for thousands of years, and perhaps it was time to reconnect with the feeling of walking on the earth and being mindful about her feet.

Just like anything regarding diet and weight-loss, we all want someone else to explain how to fix muscles and stature. The first step should be to notice how it feels to live within our own skin. This is especially important when we are recovering from an illness or injury.

After an injury, many students ask me what they can do to get back to full health *immediately*. My reply is always the same—don't *do* anything! At least not right away. The body needs time to recover. And usually the best way to do this is to allow actual *time* for healing. Why is this so hard to do? Because most of us feel like taking time off makes us seem weak. We feel the need to recover and rehabilitate as quickly as possible. We feel like this says something about the strength of our character. The faster we get back to normal exercise, the more dedicated and in control we are.

In some situations, moving quickly is truly important—such as recovery from a stroke or reconnecting a limb. It is important to reconnect nerve endings and get energy moving again as quickly as possible. But most injury is due to inattention to the moment and unawareness of space; we fall or twist or move the wrong way and something unexpected happens. Or, we've had the flu for a week and haven't kept up with our daily exercise routines. We must let go of our egos, which drive us to push through the pain.

Listen to what your body needs. Then you'll know when it's time to become active again. It'll happen one amazing morning when you wake up and just can't sit still because you know that today is the day to dance! But it is so hard to recognize when to be strong and when to be soft. We are so used to existing in a constant state of contraction that we can't let go of the tension we hold. We say we want to release tension and stress, yet we don't know what will happen if we do.

At the end of yoga class, I have all the students take a nice, deep breath and exhale on a sigh. After one of my classes, a student had tears in her eyes. "I can't do it," she said, "because if I sigh, I'll fall apart—that's how it feels." She recognized that the tension we hold within our statures seems to hold us up. She was afraid that if she sighed, if she became too soft, she would lose that thread of tension that holds her together. It took time and patience, but she was finally able to sigh a little bit at a time and truly begin to experience relaxation.

Everyone relaxes and activates at different levels. Even members of the same family have unique qualities that make the complexity of their mind-body-spirit connection completely different from everyone else's. That is why no single diet, exercise, or learning program is perfect for everyone. Each individual is a different instrument within the symphony, and no two instruments are tuned the exact same amount.

Think of the way a violinist tunes his violin. I always wondered why it had to be tuned every time it was played, even if it was only a few moments from the last time. Doesn't tuning last for a while? A cellist friend of mine explained the need for constant tuning. The instrument only plays for the moment. Everything goes into the tuning: the temperature of the room, the altitude, the humidity, the time of day, the strength of his fingers, the feel of the wood, the combination of the moment. This is why the instrument has to be tuned each time before it's played—because each moment is new and different.

Erich Schiffman, a renowned yoga teacher, reflects that the mind-body-spirit connection works the same way. We are all like a violin, or a viola, or a cello—depending on the sound we want to make. "If you were tuning a violin string, for example, you would turn the key just the right amount—not too much, not too little—in order to adjust the string tension and create the perfect sound. How much you'll turn the key cannot be known in advance. It all depends on the sound."[7]

We are all in charge of identifying our own perfect tuning. While many students look to me for answers to their mind-body-spirit connection, I simply reply, "Yoga is the yoke or union of the mind, body, and spirit. But it's not *my* mind and *your* body, it is *your* mind and *your* body." Making this connection is a personal journey to find out what is right for you and only you.

NOTES

1. "What Were the New Year's Resolutions Like in 1890–91, BodyPositive, accessed March 1, 2009, http://www.bodypositive.com/images/Toothin2.gif.

2. "Intuitive Eating to Treat Eating Disorders at Center for Change," Kim Passamore, http://www.centerforchange.com/articles/intuitive_ eating.php?c=91.

3. Ibid.

4. "Intuitive Eating: Relearning How to Eat for Life," Rebekah Mardis, accessed February 15, 2009, http://www.centerforchange.com/articles/relearning.php?c=91.

5. "Dieting Is Out," Alice Covey and Kim Passamore, accessed February 4, 2009, http://www.centerforchange.com/ articles/dieting_is-out.php?c=89.

6. Hennes

7. Erich Schiffmann, *Yoga: The Spirit and Practice of Moving into Stillness* (New York: Pocket Books, 1996), 26.

6 | IT'S ALL GOOD!

I AM OF THE OPINION THAT ALL PHYSICAL ACTIV-ity that is enjoyable, life-enhancing, and "legal" should be applauded. Many people have become sedentary shells of their true selves, and this dilemma needs to change. We all need to embrace the joy of feeling comfortable and vibrant within our own skin again!

Yet we live in a culture of one-size-fits-all in our approach to health and fitness—most recently, this approach focuses on aerobics and cardio exercise. The most common question I get about yoga is this: "Does yoga give me the aerobics and cardio workout that I need?"

I have been faced with this question hundreds of times and have spent a lot of time trying to define my position on the subject. I've defended yoga as an equal alternative to traditional aerobics and cardio workouts. I've taught that yoga can definitely increase the heart rate and keep it within levels identified by cardio guidelines if the student puts forth the effort during class. I've argued that there can be nothing more aerobic than the practice of deep breathing—the term aerobic means "with air" or "with oxygen."

Over the years, I've spent countless hours researching the aerobic and cardio benefits of yoga. I felt anxious and concerned because I had been unable to definitively express and support what I knew in my heart was a true reality of practicing yoga. I could talk until I was blue in the face about the benefits of yoga, yet it seemed as if I could never accurately convey my thoughts.

It wasn't until I began to really explore the concept of cardio exercise and its results that the light-bulb went on and I found an answer for my distress. I realized that I had been approaching the question from the wrong direction. It was a discussion between my dad and my aunt that caused me to rethink my approach.

My aunt was coming to visit and wanted directions to my house. She was familiar with the general area, so as I gave her directions, I discussed certain landmarks that would coincide with things she was already familiar with. These directions were simple and straightforward. My father was much more familiar with the area and knew that there was a faster way to get to my house. He tried to give my aunt alternate directions, which seemed simple to him and would make the journey quicker. Unfortunately, she was unfamiliar with the route he was describing, so the directions made no sense.

She had a picture in her mind of what he was describing and commented that she thought his directions would end up in the wrong place. The mental picture his directions had created for her was not the same as the actual route because she had mistaken some of the landmarks for other areas of town.

At the end of my aunt's visit, she followed my dad back to her house using the route he had described, and she finally realized where the discrepancies in opinion existed. She also reminded him that, although his route was a little quicker, both routes got her to the desired destination, and perhaps she liked the original route just as much—depending on the day.

I realized then that I was trying to force the concept of yoga into the mold of cardio. I was trying to use the same criteria for both and compare the two within the framework of only one idea. I knew the destinations of both yoga and cardio were the same, but I had forgotten that the routes were significantly different and not meant to be identical. Cardio exercise has never claimed to be yoga, so why should we compare yoga to cardio exercise? They both offer the same benefits, which can be seen in the results they create and how these results impact our lives.

I realized I had been trying to fit the proverbial square peg into a round hole. Who cares what approach we use as long as it creates a more vibrant and healthy life? Perhaps the answer to the question of why yoga is compared to cardio and aerobic exercise goes back to the discussion between my father and my aunt.

In Western culture, we've been told that there is only one route to cardiovascular health. If we don't use that route, we're only fooling ourselves, and we won't get to our destination. Those who advocate strongly for aerobic and cardio exercise try to lay exclusive claim to cardiovascular health benefits and, through ignorance, society has let them convince everyone this is true.

Let's address the issue head-on and get ready for another point of contention. There are so many opposing views on how to stay healthy, it's no wonder people are confused and constantly seeking external answers. As stated earlier, what was healthy and acceptable a few years ago is now harmful to us. Just look at the way we used to approach aerobics classes.

During the Jane Fonda era, students jumped and bounced through an hour of high-impact activity. They ended up with countless foot, knee, and hip problems. Today, low impact is finally considered key to maintaining good health, but many gym students continue to beat up their bodies through extreme exercise.

Exercise should renew, not deplete the body! Isn't the job of exercise to enhance life? Exercise is a "condiment" to life, not life itself—at least not for most people. So why do we attend classes that work us so hard we can barely walk out the door? What is the rest of the day like? In an effort to gain the prize of whatever fitness goal we may have set, other aspects of life may suffer due to lack of energy and time.

Let's look at some popular beliefs. As I said before, the word aerobic means "with oxygen." The idea is to find ways to send more oxygen to large muscle groups to be used as fuel. When we participate in aerobic exercise, we strengthen large muscles as well as the heart and lungs. This is referred to as cardiorespiratory fitness.

Cardiorespiratory fitness leads to more stamina and better movement ability. Maximal oxygen uptake (VO2max) measures how efficiently the body is able to take in oxygen, move it throughout the bloodstream, and utilize it by muscles. The more fit a person is, the higher VO2max he will be able to score. We all need strong muscles, hearts, and lungs to comfortably and actively sustain life. It's only for the past forty years, however, that this activity has occurred in structured aerobic and cardio exercise.

Cardio exercise is any activity that elevates our heart rates to a certain percentage of our maximum heart rate capabilities to help strengthen our heart muscles. In the mid–1960s, Dr. Kenneth H. Cooper started work on what he termed "aerobic exercises."[1] Dr. Cooper designed aerobic exercises for astronauts and air force pilots to combat the effects of space and lack of gravity on muscle tissue. These principles showed promising results of improved heart health for all types of heart patients.

Soon, many people began adapting aerobic exercises for the general public because they were viewed as the pinnacle of health and fitness. Today, aerobic and cardio exercises have become the norm. But let's ask ourselves this: when was the last time we went into space?

Past generations never participated in formalized aerobic or cardio exercises. Most of the world today still depends on the movement and work of completing daily tasks for its exercise. In some countries, the population dances or otherwise embraces life in ways that Western cultures have forgotten.

Why is that? Are Americans the only ones who know how to be healthy? Hardly. In fact, the United States is often considered the most obese nation in the world.[2]

My grandfather used to work with racehorses and on cattle ranches. He was very active and often achieved an elevated heart rate, which kept him healthy and active. He never went to a gym.

Not once has a doctor instructed me to raise my

heart rate. Usually, it is quite the opposite. Although cardio exercise may lower your resting heart rate, doesn't it seem a little counterintuitive to artificially speed up the heart rate in order to slow it down?

In his book entitled *Spark: The Revolutionary New Science of Exercise and the Brain*, Dr. John J. Ratey embraces and advocates the beneficial nature of running for brain health. According to him, we are born to run.

> The genes that govern our bodies today evolved hundreds of thousands of years ago, when we were in constant motion, either foraging for food or chasing antelope for hours and days across the plains. Today, of course, there's no need to forage and hunt to survive. Yet our genes are coded for this activity, and our brains are meant to direct it. Take the activity away, and you're disrupting a delicate biological balance that has been fine-tuned over half a million years.[2]

We can assume this is what people were doing half a million years ago. But what about just five thousand years ago? What if someone was a fisherman on a small island where there were no antelope? Does that mean that because he didn't run after his dinner he wasn't really part of the optimum human gene pool? I guess the ability to sustain a healthy heart and set of lungs by diving in deep water doesn't really count.

What about the goatherd who lived high in

the mountains with nowhere to run? Of course, he probably had great lung capacity due to the altitude, which was higher than the plains, but that doesn't really matter. What if his mode of survival was to set traps or depend totally on foraging? Is there no room in the optimum function of a healthy body for something other than running?

If I recall my history correctly, everyone in ancient populations had different jobs. Not every person was a runner. The best runners would chase the antelope toward the best spear-throwers, who would then bring down the animal. Then the best cooks would prepare the food, and the best tanners would use the skin to make tents and other items. As I remember from studying history, everyone in the population did what they were best at, and each job was just as important as every other job. I can only assume that not everyone ran after antelope.

But according to Dr. Ratey, we must run, even all-out sprint, in order to push the brain into maximum productivity and fully benefit from the endorphin "rush" that accompanies this type of activity. He cites studies that identified differences in lab rat brain composition when separated into active and sedentary groups as support for his firm belief that running is the optimal activity for brain health. These studies provide many important details into the increased functions and health of the brain when there is activity, and they help to recognize the importance of the brain-body connection.[4]

This is great news for all the runners out there! But what if someone isn't a runner? Ratey's book is 293 pages long, only two pages of which he devotes to what he considers "non-aerobic activity." Remember, aerobic means "with oxygen," and the most oxygen-intensive thing you can do is breathe deeply, which happens to be one of the main focuses of yoga. Imagine that! Ratey states:

> I haven't devoted much space to the discussion of non-aerobic exercise because, frankly, there is very little research into how it affects the brain in terms of learning, mood, anxiety, attention, and the other issues I've covered. It's difficult to get rats to pump iron or do yoga, so scientists are restricted to studying humans, which means they can't biopsy brain tissue after the experiments. They have to rely on blood samples and behavioral tests, which leave much more room for interpretation.[5]

In other words, people must ignore the massive amounts of data accumulated over decades that haven't been gathered in a Western laboratory, regardless of the prevalence and significance of such information. This is an interesting requirement from an associate professor of psychiatry. Where would society be if it applied this logic to the psychiatric community?

Don't misunderstand my concern—I thoroughly

enjoyed and supported the findings in Dr. Ratey's book. I truly believe in the brain-body connection and the importance of activity that elevates endorphin release and neurotransmitter enhancement. I merely wish to point out that reasonable minds can differ; knowledgeable people can disagree on paths to follow.

For example, Peg Jordan, in her book *The Fitness Instinct* says:

> What is fitness, anyway? . . . If you had to run down your food, chasing rabbits . . . fitness would imply the ability to sprint like a cheetah every other day. If you earned your daily keep by diving for sponges, you would be fit only if you could hold your breath for three minutes. Keeping up a level of fitness that exceeds your present daily activity requires an artificial overlay of exercise.[6]

Does this mean people shouldn't exert themselves if they have a desk job? Absolutely not! I hope there is more to daily life for every person than sitting at a desk. *Everyone* needs to move—it's what keeps people alive and vibrant. But lives aren't completely about movement either. Professional endurance athlete and author Mark Sisson questions these beliefs as well. "I think it's more important to eat, move, and live according to how humans are designed and not according to society's artificial developments of the last 100 years."[7] Sisson agrees with Ratey—looking at the evolutionary history of humans is the key to health—but Sisson comes to vastly different conclusions than Ratey.

> Unfortunately, the popular wisdom of the past 40 years—that we would all be better off doing 45 minutes to an hour a day of intense aerobic activity—has created a generation of over-trained, underfit, immune-compromised exerholics. Hate to say it, but we weren't meant to aerobicize at the chronic and sustained high intensities that so many people choose to do these days.[8]

Recent studies have identified a link between over-exercising the heart muscle and some forms of cardiac hypertrophy (increased heart size). This increased emphasis on cardio exercise has raised concerns regarding other cardio disease as well. In his book, *Exercise and Sports Cardiology*, Paul Thompson brings to light many of the risks associated with excessive exercise, including sudden cardiac death and acute myocardial infarction. "The acute cardiovascular adjustments to exercise provide a plausible link between exercise and these cardiovascular complications."[9]

While improving the strength of the heart through activity and exertion has always been an important part of good health, the single-minded approach of modern exercise often takes this exertion to obsessive levels. Dr. Dean Ornish adds his voice to this concern. "The risk of exercise is in direct proportion to its intensity, so moderate exercise conveys most of the benefits while decreasing the risk."[10]

As stated earlier, society has adopted the idea that if a little is good, a lot must be better. But other studies claim that a little exercise can go a long way. Dr. Steven Blaire studied 10,224 men and 3,120 women to determine how their fitness levels impacted death rates. He initially had participants perform treadmill testing and then divided them into five groups from least fit (group 1) to most fit (group 5).

As you can imagine, the death rates of the least fit (group 1) were three times greater than the most fit (group 5). The most interesting finding, though, was that the greatest differences in the impact of physical fitness existed between groups 1 and 2. The differences in health and life span between the mildly fit (group 2) and the most fit (group 5) were minimal. In other words, the benefits of fitness varied drastically among completely sedentary individuals and mildly active individuals, but benefits between mildly active individuals and extremely active individuals were statistically minimal and may even have been due to chance. "Walking thirty minutes a day (the activity level of group 2) reduced premature death almost as much as running thirty to forty miles a week (the activity level of group 5)."[11]

Dr. Ralph Paffenbarger of Stanford University found that if you burn about 2,000 calories per week, you would live about one to two years longer than a sedentary person. "The problem is that over the course of your adult life, you would need to spend about one and a half years running to live one to two years longer."[12] It's a draw! Well, actually not; because the people who didn't run the additional one and a half years spent more time with their families, therefore increasing longevity due to the happiness factor.

So where does this leave us? Should we all run or not? Do we need to push our heart rates up, or should we only incorporate moderate activity? What's the right answer? We tend to buy into the concept that if it is good for one person, it must be good for everyone. It's time to step back and ask yourself *why* you believe this. Then it's time to open an internal dialog to see what works for you.

I used to love running and I did lots of aerobics. Now, I teach and practice yoga exclusively. Does this mean that I only believe in yoga? No. It means that I have found intuitively that yoga is what is right for me at this point in my life. For me, this shift happened slowly, over the course of a few years, and continues every day. Others around me still love to run, and that is where they are comfortable today. I think this is great!

I'm not proposing that any of us give up all of our exercise and health beliefs. Just look at them more closely. Should you run ten miles a day? If you love it, go for it! If you hate it, why do it? Does your situation in life require that you hone the ability to chase down a deer on the open plain for food? Not usually. Why, then, do we feel the need to exercise as if this was our goal? It's time to be actively involved with the requirements of life and recognize that different circumstances require different approaches.

If we look at our personal habits, we'll see a pattern of the one-size-fits-all mentality. Not only do we approach exercise and diet with this mindset, we approach every aspect of life this way.

The benefits of doing cardio and aerobic activity are numerous, and most people are familiar with them. Among other things, these benefits include increased mobility, movement, and engagement of large muscle groups; increased lung capacity; increased heart rate to move oxygen to muscles; increased HDL (good cholesterol) levels; lower blood pressure; increased endurance; and weight loss. We achieve these benefits by increasing heart rates for a sustained period of time.

The cardio platform for increasing heart rate varies to include running, biking, swimming, hiking, gym classes in aerobics, treadmills, stair-climbers, elliptical machines, and so on. Basically, the principle is to get the heart rate up for an extended period of time, to quicken the breathing pattern, and to sweat. Yoga creates these same benefits, but in a different way. Pick almost any study on cardio and aerobic exercise and compare the benefit results with a similar study on yoga and they will be almost identical. In his article, "Yoga and Cardiovascular Function," Andrew Thomas speaks directly to the subject of what individuals are doing to their hearts through exercise. He suggests that people may have blindly accepted the concept that hard exercise, such as running, automatically strengthens the heart muscle and improves circulation. Thomas then goes on to explain the physiology of the heart and the role of the fascial structure.[13]

The fascia is what holds our internal structures together—it is a binding agent. Have you ever prepared chicken for a meal and removed the skin? The thin, filmy membrane that holds the skin to the chicken is called fascia. The heart is not merely sitting inside the chest cavity; it is actually connected and suspended in a complex web of this fascia that can stretch and pull on the heart muscle.

The heart, lungs, and diaphragm are all connected in this system. The diaphragm is the muscle that helps create breathing. As a person takes deep breaths, the diaphragm draws down to open the lungs. This action also creates a wonderful stretch on the heart muscle. It's like a self-massaging mechanism. While traditional forms of cardio exercise create a "pumping" contraction effect on the heart, yoga postures, which encourage deep breathing as the body stretches and bends, create a lengthening and massaging effect on the heart. In his article, Thomas identifies the physiological differences between yoga, cardio, and aerobic exercises. He explains that while cardio strengthens the cardiovascular system by forcing the heart to exert and contract rapidly, thus enlarging the heart muscle, yoga approaches cardiovascular health from the premise of utilizing the internal structure of the entire torso to stretch, massage, and lengthen the heart muscle.

I like to compare these two approaches with the differences between body builders and martial artists. Bodybuilders are continually contracting muscles in a concentric motion (toward the middle of the muscle). The focus is on building big, bulging muscle tissue that moves toward the "belly" of the muscle and away from the joints.

Martial artists, on the other hand, work to strengthen the entire length of the muscle through long, lean muscle engagement, which supports joint and skeletal structure.

The desired results of each type of activity may be strength, but the approaches are completely different. If you are looking for an increase in total mass, weight lifting and bodybuilding—muscle fiber breakdown and scar tissue buildup, resulting in the creation of bulk—will be more appealing. If, on the other hand, you are looking for functional strength and total body health and integration through the building of supple, flexible muscle fibers, I would argue that martial arts would be more fitting.

The contrast between yoga and cardio exercise is similar. We can strengthen the heart muscle by building and enlarging the muscle tissue through excessive exertion, or we can strengthen the heart muscle by stretching and lengthening the muscle tissue to keep it vibrant and active.

It is important to mindfully contemplate what your goal is when you incorporate physical activity into your life. When I was an aerobics instructor, I used to say that I wanted to look like I was twenty until I was forty. By the time I was twenty-eight, though, I was becoming "old" as an aerobics instructor.

As I moved toward practicing yoga, an amazing shift took place in my philosophy. Instead of trying to look like I was twenty until I was forty, I now wanted to be able to stand tall and feel active within my own skin until I was a hundred! I wanted to enjoy my *whole* life—not just my youth. My focus shifted from "fitness" to "health."

Dr. Ornish states: "Exercise will make you fit, but fitness and health are not synonymous. Exercise alone is not enough to make you healthy. The World Health Organization defined health as 'a state of complete physical, mental, and social well-being, not merely the absence of disease or infirmity.' "[14]

It's important to keep in mind the secondary consequences when doing any physical activity. In other words, what are the side effects of what you are doing?

For example, I taught step aerobics for many years, which started in the late 1980s as a rehabilitation exercise for knee injuries. Ironically, my knees were constantly inflamed and painful as a secondary consequence of doing step aerobics.

Many step aerobics students have suffered similar results from overuse and lack of full range of motion on the knee joints. Another area of prominent secondary consequences stems from running and high-impact aerobics. Foot, knee, and hip injuries are frequently associated with both of these activities. So, people use cardio and aerobics to improve their cardiovascular health, but they have to find additional programs to rehabilitate from the problems these activities cause.

Yoga, on the other hand, provides the cardiovascular health we're looking for and has also become a prominent rehabilitation tool to recover from secondary consequences of cardio and aerobic overexercise. Yoga is a total-life approach to health and wellness, not merely a physical approach that happens to have heart and brain benefits.

Yoga concentrates on all aspects of the mind-body-spirit connection. Yoga practitioners have recognized for years that there is more to the dimensions of health than just physical activity and altered diet. There is a real mind-body-spirit connection that we must identify and acknowledge if we want to achieve optimum health and well-being.

Wisdom is the key to incorporating any approaches that may benefit our well-being, regardless of where they originate. Unfortunately, the fitness and diet industry ignores and diminishes concepts that are not considered "Western" approaches to activity and health.

Due to the wealth and progress of our nation, many Americans no longer rely on daily physical labor for their subsistence. But the problem is that in the effort to become healthier, many of us rely on artificial ways to improve this physical component of life. For example, we may seek artificial activity in a gym setting. "Most fitness trainers will put you through a regimen based on metered progression—you must increase either repetitions, sets, intensity, or speed over time. But life is not lived as an endless linear expansion. Nowhere in nature is this concept carried out. Our normal cycles consist of energized periods, fatigue, lapses of illness, recovery, and so on."[15]

So, who should we listen to? The trainer at the gym? The expert on television? The celebrity in the magazine? How about ourselves? What a novel idea! You are your own best trainer, your own expert, maybe even your own celebrity. Should everyone move and be active—absolutely! How should this be done? I don't know! Why don't you ask yourself what you would like to do? What is your passion? Is there a way to incorporate more passion into your physical activity? Is there a way to incorporate more of your passion into life in general? The only way to find out is to be present, listen, and then move!

NOTES

1. Kenneth Cooper. *Aerobics*. New York: Bantam Books, 1969.

2. "Health Statistics: Obesity (Most Recent) by Country," NationMaster, accessed March 4, 2009, http://www.nationmaster.com/graph/hea_obe- health-obesity.

3. John J. Ratey, *Spark: The Revolutionary New Science of Exercise and the Brain* (New York: Little, Brown and Company, 2008), 248–49.

4. Ibid.

5. Ibid.

6. Peg Jordan, *The Fitness Instinct: the Revolutionary New Approach to Healthy Exercise that is Fun, Natural, and No Sweat* (Pennsylvania: Rodale Press, 1999).

7. "A Case Against Cardio (From a Former Mileage King), *Mark's Daily Apple: Primal Living in the Modern World*, Accessed February 15, 2009, http://www.marksdailyapple.com/case-against-cardio.

8. Ibid.

9. Paul D. Thompson, *Exercise and Sports Cardiology* (New York: McGraw-Hill, 2001), 128.

10. Dean Ornish, *Dr. Dean Ornish's Program for Reversing Heart Disease* (New York: Random House, 1990).

11. Ibid, 324.

12. Ibid, 327.

13. Andrew P. Thomas, "Yoga and Cardiovascular Function," *The Journal of The International Association of Yoga Therapists* 4, no. 1 (1993): 39–42.

14. Ornish, 326.

15. Jordan, 4.

7 | CHANGE YOUR WORDS; CHANGE YOUR WORLD

L ANGUAGE, ESPECIALLY OUR CONNECTION TO IT, is so interesting! If someone sees the word *read*, it could be a command to open a book now or a comment on a past perusal of a book. Context defines words. Our personal context comes from our individual history. We connect meaning to words according to our own experience and tend to slowly eliminate alternate meanings until we have a narrowly defined context of words.

In the exercise industry, instructors often use words and phrases without thought, which often has an impact on their students. During classes, instructors use verbal cues to teach students how to move a certain way. They say, "Shift your weight to one foot." "Place all your weight forward into your toes," and so on. Teachers unconsciously repeat words and phrases they have heard numerous times before. Sometimes, they aren't even aware of what they're saying or why they're saying it.

Because words hold so much meaning, it is important to be aware of what we say and how we use our words. Working at CFC has helped me to be extremely mindful of how words can affect our interactions with each other. I quickly realized that I couldn't use the typical cues for movement among the eating disorder population. Common cue words like "weight," "hips," "butt," and similar words can trigger negativity, which inhibits the mind-body reconnect. After all, one result of an eating disorder is to "not feel" the body.

Changing my teaching cues to a more anatomical vocabulary soon proved to be an amazing teaching tool. Instead of "hips," I say "hip bone" or "iliac crest." Instead of "butt," I specify "gluteal muscles" or "sits bones." Instead of "weight," I say "energy." This last one was probably the most important change. It just sounds nicer when someone tells you, "Shift all your energy into your left foot," instead of, "Shift all your weight into your left foot." I use these cues in all my classes, not just at CFC. Being aware of everyone's need for safe and supportive language helps avoid miscommunication and misunderstanding.

Miscommunication doesn't just result from the actual words used; rather, the internal context of one person may be different from another person's internal context. When we are open and objective about our words and refrain from judging someone else's use of words, we are able to create honest communication. When we are open to the idea that not everyone uses words in the same way, we move toward acknowledging the uniqueness of each individual.

I first recognized contextual miscommunication and disconnect when I introduced self-directed movement to my classes. One week, I decided to focus all my yoga classes on our ability to acknowledge and express what is happening inside our bodies. I quickly saw a lack of understanding when I asked my students to listen to what their bodies were saying. I moved the students into specific postures and then asked them how they would like to move from there. I encouraged them to listen to what they were feeling and to carefully consider what their bodies would like to do next. I instructed them to honor what they were feeling and to act on it.

I gave them a few minutes to pay attention to what was happening inside. Then I asked them to engage in whatever movement they thought would meet their bodies' needs. Almost every student in the class looked at me with a confused expression. I finally offered the students a few postures to choose from to complete their practice.

After a few classes with this same reaction, I came to the conclusion that my words and intentions were getting lost in translation. So, I spoke to the unspoken and asked the students if they understood what I wanted them to do.

It soon became apparent that many students had no idea how to listen to their bodies, let alone how to act upon what they discovered. It was hard for students to verbalize what they were feeling—they had never described their body's feelings in actual words. In fact, they often ignored what they were feeling. As hard as it was for students to verbalize their physical feelings, they were at a total loss as to what to do next. When I gave them permission to take a few minutes and do what their body wanted to do, they had no idea what to do or how to do it! They had become such a community of followers and mimics that they were no longer able to move without instruction or habitual pattern. Because the physical body has been robbed of a voice, the mind-body-spirit connection has been robbed of a language.

I decided to focus on bringing back honest and mindful language to the experience of life. I wanted to teach a class at CFC about the concept that our historical connection to words often leads us into cycles of unproductive or unhealthy behavior. I came up with the concept of the Synonym Game. First, pay attention to the words you use to describe your thoughts and emotions. Next, identify what those words really mean to you and see if they have the same meaning to the others in the class. Finally, mindfully select words that convey the same meaning but with less of a negative emphasis. Words only receive meaning from the thoughts and emotions behind them. If we truly want to change our world, all we have to do is start changing our words.

After discussing this idea with my students, we decided to actually create a synonym search for some emotional words we use in our daily lives. I brought out my computer and we began with the word "hate." That pretty much gives us nowhere to go, right? Well, maybe not. Here is the synonym string we created using the word processor on the computer:

Hate; Disgust; Aversion; Dislike; Detest; Despise; Spurn; Reject; Discard; Remove; Eliminate; Reduce; Ease; Relieve; Help; Assist; Support.

Wow, we started with hate and ended with support! How did that happen? It was simple, really. We mindfully changed our words.

The students brought up the point that at each selection, we purposely chose a nicer word. My reply: "Why *shouldn't* we try to choose nicer words? Wouldn't that make all the difference in the world?" If we could only see that when our current emotions are crying "hate," our future self may look back and find some "support" from the situation. Change a word, change your world. Another way to bring about change is to identify words, thoughts, and emotions that are closely linked to our historical experience. It is important to break the habit of negative connection.

I stumbled upon the idea of this change after a trip to San Francisco. I planned on simply canceling my classes during the week I'd be gone, but some of the CFC patients asked if they could create their own class one evening, which would be monitored by staff. I was hesitant at first. Many eating disorder patients attach the concept of exercise to their disorder. Over-exercising and ignoring body cues can play a prominent role in eating disorder activity. But after discussing how we could create a patient-led class that would be therapeutic and fun, we came up with an outline for the class, along with participation rules and guidelines.

When I returned from San Francisco, we had a therapy session where we discussed and processed the outcome of the class. Many patients were excited to share their experiences. "I found myself really listening to what I was able to do and when I started to overdo." "I remembered why I love to move and realized it doesn't have to be connected to my eating disorder." "It felt good to experience all kinds of movement in a safe and supportive environment."

We discussed the idea of relearning to trust our bodies and honor our abilities without pushing too hard. Some patients were concerned about relying on their own intuition. They weren't sure if they were ready to trust in themselves. I pointed out that we move at our own pace and reinforced the idea that we should really listen to our internal cues. The most important idea that came out of this processing session was the need to break the strangle-hold that eating disorders had attached to exercise.

I realized that exercise has not only been hijacked by eating disorders, the word "exercise" has been hijacked by our current culture. What comes to mind when you hear the word "exercise?" Whether they have an eating disorder or not, most people think of a rigid, structured, demanding program enforced and imposed upon the body for the purpose of either losing weight or gaining strength. How awful does that sound?

At the end of this processing session, I asked the class if they would be willing to commit to change the word "exercise" to the word "movement." What do you think of when I say the word "movement?" Doesn't it sound fluid and free? Doesn't it sound easy and alive? It can mean whatever we want it to. It encompasses exercise as well as all other forms of simple living—gardening, hiking, you name it. Movement implies doing, not just being.

So, we committed to change the word "exercise" to the word "movement," and thus we began to change the world. What words need changing in your life? What words need to be rediscovered? Too often, society gets so caught up in a single meaning of a word that it has strangled the vibrant life out of it. Before we know it, we're denying the ability of words to have multiple meanings, and then we wonder why there is so much miscommunication in the world.

A great example of this is the word "sensuous." What immediately comes to mind when you hear that word? Do you stop to think that sensuous has to do with the intake of information from all the senses? Or did you automatically confuse *sensuous* with "sensual," which relates to intimacy? Isn't it sad that society has allowed the meaning of such an important word to become so narrow?

Another perfect example is the word "feeling." Ask a woman how she is feeling, and she will say she is happy or sad. Ask a man, and he will say his big toe hurts. And then the woman gets mad because she thinks the man is making fun of her and not taking the conversation seriously. Well, in my opinion, the man is actually closer to being right than the woman. *Feeling* is what is physically happening inside each of us; *emoting* is the use of words to describe the physical feeling.

In my yoga classes, I explain to my students that I am happy to know what they are "emoting," but when I ask them to identify what they are feeling, I am asking them to connect to the physical sensations going on inside and then to find the words to express them. This ability to acknowledge and connect with physical feeling is largely missing in today's culture. Yet it is the basis for intuitive eating *and* intuitive living.

There has been great debate about which comes first, the physical feeling or the emotional words. I support the concept that the physical feeling comes first. Our brain then interprets and matches similar past experiences to what is happening and comes up with words to describe the physical feeling. Have you ever had a "gut feeling" that something is going to happen but you don't know what it is? You recognize the physical feeling first, and then the brain puts words to it. Sometimes this happens slowly; sometimes it is instantaneous. And sometimes it is wrong.

The connection to words is made very early in life. Children are taught things like "left foot" and "right hand." There is a one-to-one correlation in the brain. Other words have multiple layers of correlation. Have you ever gotten a headache because you forgot to eat? Your first inclination may be to take some medicine to help the headache. If you think for a minute, you may recognize that the headache was brought on by not eating. But, if you aren't paying attention, you may blame someone or something else for causing the headache and never recognize the true cause of the situation.

Actions are not dictated by the word alone; they

are also dependent on the context. This idea can also be seen in that "pit-of-the-stomach" feeling mentioned above. It may be brought on by excitement, nervousness, anger, or fear. The words rely on context for correct interpretation and communication. Sometimes the feeling turns out to be something good!

Now imagine a person is taught from the time they can speak that the "pit-of-the-stomach" feeling is always associated with fear or anger. Will they be able to feel excited and happy about a surprise party if they experience that feeling? Many patients I work with encounter this problem. They are so disconnected from the physical feelings inside their bodies that, when asked to reconnect to their bodies, they make snap judgments about what is happening without mindfully analyzing the moment.

They may lump all forms of discomfort under the heading of pain and stay away from any movement that asks more of them than complete relaxation. They may also lump all feelings of fear and nervousness under the heading of anger because they haven't stopped to honestly evaluate the situation.

What if someone is taught that love is displayed by anger and abuse? Will that person be able to identify love with gentleness and care? Is it any wonder that it is so difficult to communicate with words alone? To be truly capable of sharing experiences with others, we must first understand the physical feeling behind our words. Then we can start expressing our historical context and acknowledge the historical context of others.

Words express a person's story. Words influence a person's environment. Try finding space in your life to change these words: use "fluid" instead of "flexible"; find space for the word "plentiful" instead of "hectic"; say "vibrant" and "abundant" as often as you can. Join my campaign: Change your words; change your world.

8 | SO, WHAT NOW?

WHY IS THE MIND-BODY-SPIRIT CONNECTION SO important? It's important because of what it allows us to experience. True balance and unity of all aspects of our lives only have meaning if they help us move beyond ourselves to impact the world around us.

The ego-mind, however, can sometimes get the better of everyone. The ego-mind is reflected in many forms. All of us inevitably suffer from the "-est" syndrome at some point. This is the need to be the strongest, weakest, smartest, dumbest, happiest, saddest, and so on. It might not even matter if the form of the "-est" syndrome is positive or negative, as long as someone wins the contest. In our competition to become the "-est" at something, we can get lost in the game, all in the name of doing what we think is expected—what is right "-est."

These patterns come from all walks of life and

all spiritual backgrounds. In the effort to do what is right and appropriate, many people have moved away from certain truths and become blinded by habits and traditions. Some of us continually beat our-selves up in the quest to be all things to all people. One area in which we sometimes fall prey to the "-est" syndrome is in our attempt to be the humblest. Society uses a broad brush to paint many detrimental practices with the color of humility.

This idea shows up quite strongly in the mis-conception that true selflessness must come from self-denial and self-deprecation. A woman in particu-lar may feel that in her role as wife and mother, she should ignore her own needs and downplay her health and welfare for the sake of her husband and children. If she ignores herself, she may mistakenly believe she is being selfless. This is not true.

Often, in another effort to appear selfless, women diminish and demean themselves. They speak nega-tively of their bodies and in turn give those around them permission to do the same. We feed off of one another's negative body talk in our quest to be the "-est." And then we wonder why those around us hate their own bodies!

Somewhere along the line, the Anglo-Christian world adopted the philosophy that the spirit is what makes us "good," and the body is what makes us "bad." We wrap our arms around the idea that we must condemn and subjugate the body almost to the point of self-loathing in order to feel as if we are overcoming the body and lifting the spirit out of the natural arena in which it now resides.

Many of us seek to achieve this goal to show that we can overcome the temptations and inadequacies of the body. We may feel that this is the ultimate spiritual task. But, in the effort to turn thoughts away from ourselves and toward others, we may find a backlash of consequences. As we ignore our bodies' needs, we actually create what we are most trying to ignore—we find ourselves caught up in body-consciousness.

In his book, *Yoga: The Spirit and Practice of Moving into Stillness*, Erich Schiffman describes what happens when someone falls into this trap of self-ignorance. If someone has a headache or toothache, that is where thoughts and concerns will reside. All attention will be taken up with the aches and pains that come from the dis-ease. He notes a similar problem when upkeep on a car is ignored: the driver is constantly worried about the car breaking down.[1]

This same principle applies to the body. When we ignore the health and care of our bodies, we create "body-ache" and focus all of our attention on what is wrong. We have no time or energy to focus outside of ourselves because we are caught up in the cycle of ignoring, suppressing, and denying our bodies' needs. On the other hand, when we keep our bodies in good running order, just like a car, we are able to enjoy the ride and turn our attention to the scenery outside!

When we pay mindful attention to our bodies, we start to recognize that the physical aspect of life is just as important as the mental and spiritual. We feel the zippers of the ski coat engage and find the mind-body-spirit connection, an important part of which is the internal voice. Isn't it interesting that people actively seek to overcome the negative or "bad" voices around them, and yet they give in to the negative voice within?

When we allow the negative voice within to speak loudly, we then seek for a positive external voice to balance what is happening. Have you ever said something negative about yourself, only to have those around you jump in with a positive comment? Do you vocalize the negative so that others will feel obligated to say something positive, or do you actively say positive things to others to counter the negative voice within your own self? Listen to this internal conversation!

It is important to open an honest internal dialog. In an Anglo-Christian tradition, or any other spiritual tradition, how can a person love the spirit and yet hate the body when the two are so closely connected?

How can a person love his neighbors as himself when he doesn't love himself first? I would hate to treat my neighbor with some of the thoughts that go through my head about myself. We can't live just half of this commandment. Start paying attention, and be gentle and loving from the inside out. It's time to stay awake.

Isn't it interesting that kids or pets do crazy things when they feel ignored? The solution isn't to ignore them more and talk about how bad they are; instead, pay attention and get them to connect with someone. The same is true for the mind-body-spirit connection. An individual can't ignore any one area to focus exclusively on another area—it is all connected. They are all responsible for making you uniquely you!

Nobody was meant to have the same body as someone else. How boring would that be? I am five foot four on a really good hair day. I will never be five foot ten. So I enjoy and find interest in who I am just as I am. But that doesn't mean I can abuse my body and still think I am who I should be. Just as excessive thinness through starvation is not who people truly are, excessive weight does not reflect who people truly are either. When you become truly connected to the "subtle" feeling of actually living inside your body, you will know who you should naturally be. Some of us are naturally small, and some are naturally large. So what? Actually, how amazing!

We can create peace within our spirits when we feel welcome and comfortable within our bodies. Sri Swami Satchidananda states: "We're born fine until we de-fine ourselves, and then we use these definitions to see how we are different rather than how we are alike. So now we must re-fine ourselves."[2] It is time to shift from a dialog of dissatisfaction and negative image to a lovingly mindful connection to the entire being.

Once we recognize the need to treat our bodies with kindness and gentleness, we need to recognize a second area of stress within our culture—that of thinking that we must do everything all at the same time. We need to ask ourselves, "What is there room for today?" You would never continue pouring water in a glass that is already full, yet this is exactly what people do in life.

There is a proverbial list of all the things that are designated as good and necessary, and we try to stuff more and more things into our lives until we are bursting at the seams. And then we wonder why we are under stress! I want to be a great piano player, and I know that if I practice enough I will be. This is a fabulous goal, but I also want to clean my house and visit my family. Just because something is good doesn't make it relevant. There is *not* enough room for everything at the same time. We have to give something up to get something else. Life is about choices, and the goal is to make the best choices for this particular moment.

You may have heard the story of the monkey who put his hand into a knot hole in a tree to retrieve a nut. When he closed his fist around the nut, his hand no longer fit through the hole. The monkey held on to the nut, even with a predator close by, because he didn't understand that he couldn't keep the nut and still escape.

We are like this in our own lives. We may look back and remember what we used to do or how we used to act and mourn the loss of the past. Perhaps we look to the future and idealize the time when we will have accomplished it all, when all the good routines have become habit and we don't have to try so hard—then we complain that today isn't tomorrow, when we will be more perfect.

Perhaps we look at and compare ourselves to others and find our box lacking. What we don't recognize is that we only see the "amazing" parts of other people's boxes, not the behind-the-scenes workings. Why do some people always want what they don't have? Why do some people hold on to or fantasize about the nut inside the tree?

I prefer to think the process is like rock climbing or climbing a ladder. To move to the next carabiner or rung, we must let go of the one we are connected to right now. This happens all the time in life. Children move from one grade in school to another, shoppers buy new clothes and give away the old ones. Brave individuals cut their hair or change their makeup. Yet most of us don't feel like this should apply to all areas of life. Why not?

Think of what the main focus was in your life at a younger age. How much of that applies to your adult life today? If it was so important then, why isn't it important now? It's because it is not relevant to you now. So, if your past is no longer relevant to your present (other than the wisdom you gained from those experiences), why should someone else's box be relevant to you either? It's because everyone has fallen into the cookie-cutter world of one-size-fits-all. Wouldn't it be great if we could just look at others and be in awe of their accomplishments and successes without wanting the exact same thing for ourselves? Most people spend way too much time seeking to be amazing when they should really be spending more time being amazed!

This is where the idea of becoming like a little child can really offer new meaning to life. Children are amazed at everything. They approach life with open arms and open hearts. Little children truly embrace life within their bodies. They play and explore movement without inhibition. As they get older, they are told to quit acting like a three-year-old, so they do! How sad.

As we grow up, we become constricted and inhibited in our movement and enjoyment of our healthy, active bodies. We grow tense and rigid in our physical expressions of life. When was the last time you went dancing? When was the last time you rolled around on the floor? Do you play with your toes anymore? Becoming like a child has much to do with the way we embrace life within our physical selves.

So, why is it important to reclaim and embrace this mind-body-spirit connection? At its simplest level, it's for the insight and intuitiveness this connection brings to the forefront of life. Many people identify this with being in tune with God; others may identify this with being in tune with the energy of life. Whatever you identify this process with, it is important to recognize the power of this internal voice.

A few years ago, I spoke to a woman's group on the topic of becoming in tune with ourselves so that we can then become more in tune with the needs of those around us. Using the example of sunlight streaming through a window, I related the importance of listening to personal intuition through becoming still.

Have you ever been near a window when the sunlight is shining and, instead of looking out the window, looked sideways at the rays of light as they come into the room? If you pay close attention, you can see the dust particles refracted in the sunlight. Why don't we see this all the time? The dust particles are always there, and the sunlight is there many times also.

What you experienced in that particular moment was the mindfulness and stillness of awareness. Stillness allows us to become more aware of our surroundings, and mindfulness allows us to become more tuned in to subtle experience.

It is the same concept as thinking that the phone is about to ring, and then it does. Have you ever wondered how this works? It's simple, really. It is a law of physics and elements. Everything in the universe is made up of energy. Each type of energy—light waves, sound waves, heat waves, and so on—has a different wavelength. Our bodies react to the waves of energy around us. The stronger the wave, the easier it is to notice—like loud music. The more subtle the wave, the harder it is to notice, but it is still there.

When the phone is about to ring, an electrical current vibrates through the receiver of the phone. If it is very quiet, and if you are in tune with the subtleness of the moment, your body will actually feel the vibration before you hear the sound. Your subconscious brain recognizes the wave of energy as being associated with the phone ringing, and so you get the feeling that the phone is about to ring. Isn't that amazing?

This is how personal intuition and insight work. Like the dust particles, insight is always there, just waiting for us to be still and tune in. But we've been programmed to only listen to the loud and obvious. This is why the adage, "the squeaky wheel gets the grease" is so prominent in the world.

Society has encouraged us to push through pain

and ignore natural instincts; to speak up and be heard at all times, regardless of right or wrong; to fight for a "piece of the pie." Many individuals have lost the ability and even the desire to listen to the subtle, intuitive part of themselves. They are waiting for external information to guide them to the important things in life. They have become simply robots of habits and external cues; they have lost the basic ability to interact with and notice others.

Too often, we are so fixed on the loud voices or the obvious needs around us that we have no time to *be still* and simply listen for the quiet distress emanating from the ones closest to us. We are so busy checking off the items on our daily to-do list that we have no time to sit quietly and seek peace.

We all say we want peace and stillness, but at the same time we condemn ourselves for taking a moment out of our hectic lives because we feel as if we are being lazy or unproductive. When was the last time you took a nap? Did you feel guilty when you did? When was the last time you meditated? Do you feel as if this falls into the category of idleness or laziness? If you don't ever give a true moment to stillness, how can you ever expect to get in tune with yourself or others? It is time to undo some of the habitual patterns life has fallen into.

Someone once asked the famous yoga teacher, Swami Satchidananda, "What are you, a Hindu?"

"No," he replied, "I'm an Undo. I'm trying to teach people how they can undo the patterns that cause damage to their minds and bodies so they can begin to heal."[3] Giving the self a chance to mindfully recognize unconscious habits will allow a person to strive for true happiness—true joy in life. Speaking of this quest for happiness, Swami Satchidananda states:

> Nothing can bring us lasting happiness, but we have that already if we simply quiet down the mind and body enough to experience more of an inner sense of peace, self-worth, and self-esteem, one that comes not from getting or from doing but simply from being. And the paradox and the irony is that not being aware of this, we end up running everywhere else looking for this elusive happiness, in the process disturbing the inner joy and peace we could have if we simply quieted down the mind and body enough to experience that.[4]

When we recognize this need to find a more mindful way to live, we will seek for peace and stillness. But, the hardest place to find this is within ourselves. This is where the rubber meets the road, so to speak. You may be thinking, "So what?" Or even, "So, what now?" Now, life begins—again. None of us can just let go of everything we've ever learned and everything we've ever done. Remember, change doesn't happen—shift happens.

What is my purpose in sharing this book with you? I want to help you wake up and make you question your self. It isn't enough to ask what you want. *Why* do you want it? My husband always feels like he has to walk on egg shells if I ever mention that I want to make changes in my life. He is the "goal and action word" king! He wants a set and written plan for everything— laid out step-by-step. This is a great concept sometimes, but it doesn't apply to everything. Sometimes life just requires awareness and the ability to question what will work in the moment. So ask the questions!

Do you want to lose weight? Great! Maybe. Why? Do you want to exercise more? Great! Maybe. Why? Do you want to create new habits? Great! Maybe. Why? Does this make sense? Hopefully everyone has figured out the key by now.

Life is not so much about what people do; it is more about *why* they do what they do. Ask yourself this question: "If I were living on a deserted island, would I choose to do this?" People should choose to do what they love! It doesn't work all the time. I don't think I would choose to do laundry and dishes on a deserted island. But I love a clean house, so it works! Listen to the intuitive! Listen to the connectedness within the mind-body-spirit ski coat. Don't be so sure that anyone else really has the answer that is right for everyone.

Now, for a disclaimer. There are times when the capacity to honor this truth may be diminished due to circumstances such as substance abuse, mental illness, eating disorders, and so forth. These are times when it is most important to recognize the people who will be your anchor in the storm.

Interestingly enough, the best anchors are those who have found their own mind-body-spirit connection. They are able to help others get back on track. Those who challenge others to dig deep and find their way back to self-connection make the best advocates for healing and health.

Honor the true self; embrace the true individual; connect to intuition; let external voices stay that way—external; seek what enhances life through personal experience and judgment; allow shift to happen when it is time; be present within your own skin; be amazed at every day; ask "so what?" and let it be an honest dialog, not merely a flippant response; don't be afraid to start over. Remember: every day is a new day, because every hour is a new hour, because every minute is a new minute, because every breath is a new breath. How often can we start over? With every breath! GO FORTH AND CONQUER!

NOTES

1. Eric Schiffmann, *Yoga: The Spirit and Practice of Moving into Stillness.* (New York: Pocket Books, 1996), 26.
2. Dean Ornish, *Dr. Dean Ornish's Program for Reversing Heart Disease* (New York: Random House, 1990).
3. Swami Satchidananda, as quoted by Dean Ornish.
4. Ibid.

9 | WHAT'S A DAY WITHOUT A "LEANNE-ISM?"

I PROMISED ALL OF MY STUDENTS THAT I WOULD include some of their favorite sayings and thoughts in this book. I asked each of my students to write down things that I have said over the years that have made an impact in their lives and then send them to me.

This brings to mind the old saying "be careful what you wish for." Putting my voice under a microscope has been interesting, to say the least. It has also been humbling to see my thoughts through my students' eyes. So to all my students—thank you, and I hope you don't get tired of hearing these sayings one more time! We all fall into speech and thought patterns that are uniquely ours. Here are a few of mine, as well as a few yoga and life lessons that I use quite frequently.

WHEN YOU'RE READY—JUST LET GO!

This is the inspiration for everything I do. This is a

term I first used when leading my students into seated boat posture. I instruct the students to hold on to their knees as they slowly move back into their "sit bones" and lift their feet off the floor. Then I encourage them to let go of their knees and use their core muscles to balance. I tell them when they are ready to just let go.

Over the years, I have found that this sentiment is much more of a life lesson than merely a yoga cue, so I added the phrase "Life lesson #1, according to LeAnne," and a whole new world of possibilities opened up. Letting go can signify releasing tension and stress or it can signify jumping out of an airplane to sky dive. We can't put limitations on what we will need to let go of—we can only "be ready" to do it!

JUST LET IT BE OKAY.

We judge every conscious moment or judge ourselves for not being conscious of the moment. We need to be aware of what we do and say, but we need to be more capable of letting go of our judgment of the moment. As long as we are aware, we will shift toward change. Be kind to yourself. It will happen if you just let it be okay.

IT'S JUST A PLACE TO GO.

Every time I lead a class into an "interesting" posture, I say: "Don't worry about it; it's just a place to go—like Hawaii." I use the example of going to

Hawaii because we can all relate to the idea. Some people have been there; some people are planning to go there; some people have booked the flight; some people have no desire to go to Hawaii. Yoga postures and life situations we want to achieve are like going to Hawaii. We are all in different stages of the process, but remember, there is really no magic to any single circumstance—it's just a place to go.

LISTEN TO WHERE YOU ARE IN SPACE.

What a strange idea. It is so important, though, to be connected within ourselves and with the world around us. Have you ever been in the mall or somewhere really crowded and noticed that there are always a few people who have no clue what is going on around them? They walk right into you without saying a word or butt in line without comment. I don't think they are intentionally mean or rude; I think they are just unaware of where they are in space.

It is important for us to become aware of what is present and for us try to be in tune with the moment. This helps us find and improve balance in our lives mentally, physically, and spiritually. Recognize where you are in space.

IT ALL DEPENDS ON WHERE YOU SET YOUR GAZE.

In yoga, the gaze is defined as "drishti," meaning a point for the external and internal gaze to stay connected to during postures and meditation. When we focus on a firm point, our minds become calm and stable; when our minds are stable, our bodies become calm and stable. This creates balance. So, if you want to create balance—in your body and in your life—it all depends on where you set your gaze.

IT'S ALL GOOD!

This one is a no-brainer. There is good to be found in any situation if we allow ourselves to be open to the possibilities. There are so many approaches to any given situation and so many options in any circumstance, yet we are programmed to identify choice as right and wrong. Sometimes this is true, but more often it is just a matter of right and right.

Or, perhaps, we can still find something good within the wrong path if we allow ourselves to learn from it. When we allow that there are many paths to the same goal, many right ways to accomplish the same thing, and many different things to be experienced during a single moment, we will recognize that we just need to relax and lighten up a little—it's all good!

WHOEVER SAID WE SHOULD TOUCH OUR TOES? SOMEONE WHO COULD!

I hate when my students feel like they have to conform mentally, physically, or spiritually to someone else's concept of who they should be. I try to get students to recognize that experts are only experts on what they have accomplished themselves and, therefore, they will always advocate for their own success.

They ask us to let go of what's in our box to embrace what is in their box. Just because something happens to work for someone else doesn't mean that it is right for you. It may be, but it may not be. Give ideas careful thought and honest attention, and *then* make choices that are right for you. Be careful about what others state is a goal to be desired; it may turn out to be undesirable in your life, which is just fine!

JUST SIT WITH IT.

When we try new things for the first time, we may feel uncomfortable and anxious. Our fight-or-flight instinct may lead us to try to move away from the situation without really giving it a chance. If we feel challenged in a situation, the first step is to try to relax and acknowledge what is happening. The most important part of any moment is to just sit with it for a moment.

NICE / BEAUTIFUL.

Why do we speak so negatively to ourselves? I think it's because we don't want people to think we are conceited or egotistical. The problem is that if we don't speak lovingly to and about ourselves, who will?

I try to liberally incorporate the words "nice"

and "beautiful" throughout my yoga classes instead of words like "perfect" and "good." What if some of my students notice that they aren't doing something as "perfectly" as the person next to them? Suddenly, my words could create a sense of dis-ease. Instead, I try to use words that are descriptive of the energy being conveyed, not the posture itself.

WE DON'T LIVE BECAUSE WE BREATHE; WE LIVE BECAUSE WE PAUSE.

When I was first studying to be a yoga teacher, I wanted to understand why breathing was so important to the practice. In my study of breathing techniques and the teachings of Nancy Ruby, I came to believe that we don't live because we breathe; rather, we live because we pause. There are four parts to a breathing cycle. The description I give to my students is that breathing is like riding on an elevator.

Have you ever felt an elevator move to a particular floor and then "settle" or pause for a moment before the doors open?

This is the elevator's way to connect with the new floor and create stability. Likewise, when we breathe we pause between the inhale and exhale. I like to explain that the pause after the inhale allows the body to fully absorb the oxygen and move carbon dioxide into the lungs for removal.

Then, the pause after the exhale allows the

diaphragm to relax and prepare for the next inhale. The function of the pause, while almost instantaneous, may be as beneficial as the inhale and exhale themselves. Perhaps, more important than associating this teaching with breathing, we truly do live because we pause. So take some time today to pause—and breathe.

MAKE A FIST; NOW, MAKE A FIST AGAIN!

Many of my students begin yoga as an exercise activity to build strength, and I try to guide them to question their understanding of strength and its reflection in the physical body. Some of the ideas they speak of are things like "rock hard abs" or "killer arms." These terms are usually linked to the muscle's ability to concentrically contract—pulling the belly of the muscle fibers toward the center, as in a bicep curl.

I try to teach them the true meaning of strength by asking them to make a fist as tightly as they can; then I ask them to make a fist again. The students always look confused, and then one or two of them will open their fist in order to close it again in a new contraction.

This is the lesson: in order to make a new fist, we must let go of the old contraction and engage a new contraction. Our muscles were not meant to stay in a constant state of concentric contraction, they were made to move. Relaxation and lengthening movements are as vital for strength as our ability to create a concentric contraction. To be truly strong, we must know when and how to be soft.

SPEAK TO THE UNSPOKEN.

This is, perhaps, one of the greatest lessons I have learned in yoga. Nancy Ruby taught me that we need not be afraid of addressing what is already hovering in the room. To "speak to the unspoken" is a reminder that to leave things hidden or unaddressed leads to dis-ease. It is important to never be afraid of any subject. We need to be thoughtful, careful, and honest in order to allow others to feel safe in our presence. If I, as a teacher, can move into the unspoken realm and bring it to light, this will give my students the permission and courage to speak to their own unspoken issues.

REPEAT AFTER ME: THIS IS MY BIG TOE; THIS IS MY EAR; THIS IS MY NOSE; THIS IS MY HEART.

I was teaching kid's yoga one day to a class who had brought their kids in because it was spring break. It was amazing to see the parents interact with their children as we all participated in the kid's yoga story. Everyone was smiling and active. I noticed that a few moms were showing their children which hand or foot to move.

I had to stop and smile because another lightbulb moment was happening. Many times in class I would notice that someone was having a hard time identifying which was their left or right hand or foot. I would always joke that we had learned these functions as little kids, but we never had to think about them again. Watching the parents go through these same lessons with their own children made me realize that, again, it is important to become as little children.

At the end of class, I had everyone sit on their mat in a folded leg position, and then I told them they all had to repeat after me and follow my actions. "This is a lesson to remind us about ourselves—so we don't forget," I said. Then we went through the phrase: "This is my big toe (touch our toe); this is my ear (touch our ear); this is my nose (touch our nose); this is my heart (bring our hands into prayer position above our heart)." Sometimes we forget where the heart is, and this is a good reminder—physically, mentally, and spiritually.

IT FEELS GOOD, IN A WEIRD SORT OF WAY.

Many times, we find ourselves in positions that bring new sensations to our bodies and minds. It is important to acknowledge the sensations before we try to categorize them.

Sometimes we lump all difficult sensations into the category of pain when it is really just mild discomfort. When we tell ourselves it feels good, in a weird sort of way, we can be honest and open with what is really happening.

JUST BECAUSE I CAN PUT MY FOOT AROUND MY HEAD DOESN'T MEAN I FIND IT USEFUL!

Many new yoga students are excited about trying difficult and challenging poses. Often, they want to try something within the "pretzel" family of postures. I always challenge the students to examine their reasons for wanting to tackle these poses. Usually, they like the idea of doing what they consider "hard" things because their ego-mind is still in control of their mindfulness.

I smile and tell them that just because I *can* put my foot around my head doesn't mean I do my dishes that way. Students who have studied with me for a while love this comment because it gives them permission to really contemplate why they do yoga and why they like certain poses. I encourage doing a few poses that are strictly for building up feelings of accomplishment, but I remind myself not to get so caught up in these poses that I lose the true essence of yoga.

RECOGNIZE WHAT YOU ARE FEELING, NOT JUST WHAT YOU ARE EMOTING.

I'm always interested in my students' emotions, and I am happy to listen to what they are "emoting." But when I ask them what they are "feeling," I want to know if their knee hurts or if their feet are connected to the earth. "Feeling" is about what is physically happening; "emoting" is the use of words to describe the physical feeling.

For many of us, connecting to and verbalizing what is going on inside is a very hard place to engage. If we can learn to be mindful of this difference between feeling and emoting, we can become really in tune with the subtle feelings inside us.

TAKE A NICE, DEEP BREATH AND EXHALE ON A SIGH.

Sighing is so important! It can release all sorts of tension and stress with a simple expulsion of extra "stuff" that tends to hang out as residual breath in the lungs. It's kind of like "pressure washing" your breathing cycle. It also gives us an opportunity to allow our breath to be renewed. So, take a nice, deep breath and exhale on a sigh!

IF THE ONLY THING YOU LEARN FROM ME IS TO BE MINDFUL AND STAY PRESENT, THEN I HAVE TAUGHT YOU THE ESSENCE OF YOGA.

Yoga, at its heart, isn't about poses or breathing. There are eight limbs, or *ashtangas*, within the life practice of yoga. Each limb focuses on a different area of life: abstinences, observances, movement, breath, internal focus, concentration, meditation, and inspiration. While each of them might require a separate book to understand, they all point to the same principle: life is about being mindful and present.

It doesn't matter if you are on a mat or in a car, if

you are being mindful, you are practicing yoga—you are practicing life. If you never touch your toes, so what? But if you never contemplate the journey to *try* to touch your toes, you have truly misunderstood the process.

YOGA DOESN'T DEFINE YOU—IT REFINES YOU!

We tend to speak of ourselves in terms of "I am (something)." We are really good at defining ourselves. We say, "I am strong," or, "I am flexible." What does that mean? I like to think of how this would be said in Spanish. It would translate as, "I have strength," or, "I have flexibility." Yoga is not a definition of who we are; rather, it is a mirror of how we exist in the world today. When we honestly and mindfully look at ourselves in the mirror, we will allow the negative aspects of ourselves to be acknowledged and improved.

More importantly, we will allow the positive aspects of ourselves to be simply another part of us— not the totality of who we are. Yoga reminds us that we are a whole person—a holistic person. Saying, "I am strong," no more captures the totality of who I am than saying, "I am thirsty." If we truly have a need to define ourselves, let's say, "I am alive!"

THE ENDING

At the end of every yoga class, I say the same thing. I like this continuity and security within the process. It feels like a fuzzy pair of slippers, and my students let me know if I forget the process. I end class by saying this: "Inhale your arms up; interlace your fingers; turn your palms up; look up and smile; don't let this be the last smile of your day; now, exhale, hands to your heart; thank you for sharing yoga with me. Namaste."

SOMEONE ONCE ASKED BUDDHA:
"Are you a god?"
And he replied, "no."
They asked, "Are you a prophet?"
And he replied, "no."
They asked, "Well, what are you?"
And Buddha replied,

AWAKE!

ABOUT THE AUTHOR

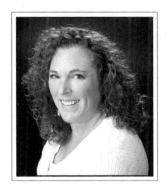

LeAnne W. Tolley has worked in the health and wellness industry for the past twenty years as a certified aerobics instructor, certified yoga teacher with Yoga Alliance, and registered yoga therapist with the International Association of Yoga Therapists. She graduated from Utah Valley University with a degree in business management and community health and is a certified health education specialist.

LeAnne also works as a yoga therapist at The Center for Change, in Orem, Utah, creating yoga as a therapy for patients with eating disorders. She focuses on helping individuals create healthy, balanced lives through "functional fluidity" and "intuitive living." She is a frequent guest speaker on diet and exercise, body image issues, and health and wellness.